AFFIRMED

AN INCLUSIVE GUIDE
TO MEDICAL AND
SURGICAL TRANSITION

DR. SIDHBH GALLAGHER, MD

Chapters

Section 1

Healthcare for Transfeminine Patients and Non-Binary Assigned Male at Birth Patients

Section 2

Healthcare for Transmasculine Patients and Non-Binary Assigned Female at Birth Patients

Dedication

This book is dedicated to all my patients past, present and future. You will never know how much I am in awe of your bravery and authenticity. Thank you for allowing me to find my life's purpose by hopefully helping you along your journey. I am truly honored by the trust you and your family members put in me every day.

I can't imagine more deeply gratifying work. Also to supportive family and friends of my patients, you have renewed my faith in humanity.

Dr G

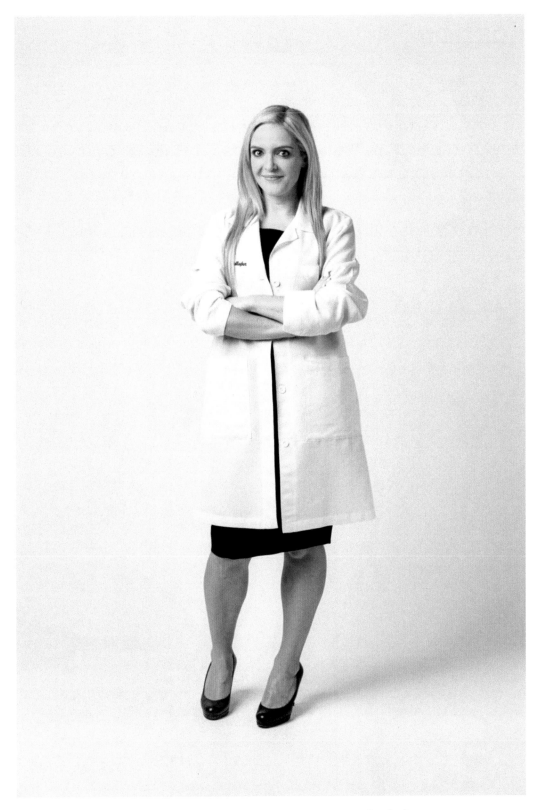

Figure 1 Dr Sidhbh Gallagher is located in Miami, Fl.

About Dr. Gallagher

Dr. Sidhbh (pronounced "Sive") Gallagher is originally from Ireland. She is a double board-certified plastic surgeon who has dedicated her career to serving the transgender and non-binary community. She became an Assistant Professor at the Indiana University School of Medicine in 2015 where she founded and directed the University of Indiana Gender Affirmation Program. There, Dr. Gallagher innovated new techniques such as Masculoplasty as well as teaching and publishing on gender affirmation surgery. Dr. Gallagher now has a busy practice in Miami, Florida where along with her sister Neasa, she takes care of patients from all over the world. For more information visit www.gallagherplasticsurgery.com Gallagher Plastic Surgery and Gallagher Med Spa are located in Miami, Fl. Phone 305 204 9598 Email; info@gallagherplasticsurgery.com

Disclaimer

This book outlines many medical treatments, procedures and also after care, however these can be hazardous without proper medical supervision. This book does not substitute for the care of a medical practitioner. Consult with your medical practitioner before engaging in any of the treatments, procedures and aftercare in this book. The authors disclaim responsibility for any adverse effects that may result directly or indirectly from information in this book. Also note knowledge and best practices in this field are constantly changing, so as new research becomes available many aspects of practice and medical treatment described in this book may also change.

Introduction

Finding accurate information to help along the path to medical and surgical transition can be challenging. There is still a lack of competent providers in this field and though the internet is a wonderful resource while transitioning, there is just too much myth and inaccuracy out there. This book was conceived in response to just that. Written by Dr. Gallagher and a group of dedicated colleagues who serve the transgender and non-binary community, it is designed to be a solid resource when it comes to transgender health care. It is primarily designed to deliver information to patients in a way that's straight forward and jargon free. These concepts can be difficult enough to understand without reading a medical dictionary at the same time! Transitioning is such a complex process and the physical aspect of it is just one part of the puzzle. Our hope is that this guide will help de-mystify the process.

Gender Dysphoria

by Dr Sidhbh Gallagher

What is gender dysphoria?

Gender dysphoria refers to discomfort or distress that is caused by a discrepancy between a person's gender identity and that person's sex assigned at birth. For many years now it has been recognized that gender dysphoria can be a severe medical condition in some cases and can be associated, with suicide. The good news is we now know that treatments for gender dysphoria can work very nicely in helping relieve it. In adults, the following features can be used to diagnose it.

Patients have 2 of the following for at least 6 months:

1. A marked incongruence between one's experienced/expressed gender and primary and/or secondary sex characteristics

2. A strong desire to be rid of one's primary and/or secondary sex characteristics

3. A strong desire for the primary and/or secondary sex characteristics of the other gender

4. A strong desire to be of the other gender

5. A strong desire to be treated as the other gender

6. A strong conviction that one has the typical feelings and reactions of the other gender

What is the difference between gender dysphoria and gender non-conforming?

Gender non-conformity just means a person's gender identity, role or how they express their gender differs from what is considered "normal" for their biological sex in a particular culture. Not all gender non-conforming individuals will experience gender dysphoria.

Sexuality is different!

A wise mental health professional once explained to me the difference between sexuality, which is who a person is attracted to and gender identity. Sexuality (being straight, lesbian, gay, bisexual) refers to who a person would like to go to bed

WITH gender identity is who a person goes to bed AS. Sexual orientation is therefore different from gender identity and they are independent of each other.

Are transgender patients mentally ill?

Experts agree that just because a person is transgender, trans-sexual or gender non-conforming does NOT mean they have a disorder. In some patients however the distress from gender dysphoria may be severe enough to meet criteria for this diagnosis.

How common is it?

It is very difficult to figure out world-wide how common it is to be transgender or gender non-conforming as obviously many cultural factors come into play. In the past we tried to figure out these numbers by looking at the numbers of patients showing up for treatment of gender dysphoria. Many patients may not want or need or have access to these treatments, so a better way is to ask the general population of people how they identify. In the USA the prevalence of a self-reported transgender identity in children,

adolescents and adults ranges from 0.5 to 1.3%.

This is much higher and more common than we had previously thought.

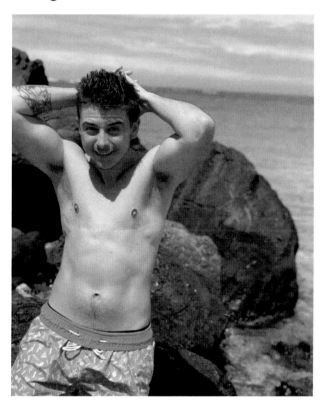

Figure 2 Maculoplasty patient Thomas

How is gender dysphoria treated?

In the second half of the 20th centaury the medical profession began to realize that gender dysphoria could effectively be relieved using approaches to help make patients more comfortable in their gender roles. As medicines improved, better and safer hormonal treatments as well as surgical techniques were developed to help patients.

A key concept in helping transgender and gender non-conforming patients is individualized care. No two patients are the same and not all patients will need or want hormones and/or surgery. Physicians now understand that it is a highly personal journey and not a "one size fits all" treatment. This is especially true with greater understanding of the non-binary community.

As such many different techniques are available to help affirm patients as much as possible. Techniques are constantly improving as more patients are getting surgery. For example, our technique of masculoplasty lets patients get their FTM top surgery without using drains, which was unheard of in the past.

Terminology

Just as gender identity is diverse there can be a broad range of terms, some culture specific and some privileged. Here are some more common terms.

Transgender - refers to the broad spectrum of individuals who sometimes temporarily or sometimes permanently identify with a gender different from their gender at birth. For example, a patient may be assigned female at birth but identify as a man- this is a transgender man, or a patient may be assigned male at birth but identify as female this is a transgender woman. A patient may identify also in some other category than the binary ideas of male or female.

Gender expansiveness - conveys a wider, more flexible range of gender identity and/or expression than typically associated with the binary gender system.

Cis-gender – refers to an individual whose gender identity is that with which they were assigned at birth.

Gender fluidity – A person's gender identity may change with time.

Intersex- Intersex people are individuals born with any of several variations in sex characteristics that do not fit the typical definitions for male or female bodies.

Humans are complex and diverse creatures the medical community now understands that there is a lot more going on than just biological sex. We also now know that especially if we are concerned for a patient's well-being and as medical professionals there is nothing more important. These other factors are especially important.

Each individual will have:

A biological sex

Sexuality- who they are attracted to (if anyone at all).

Gender expression – how the patient presents their gender to the world through clothing, appearance or other mannerisms.

Gender identity- This is ones deeply held core sense of being male or female, some of both or neither.

Each of these aspects can be independent of each other.

Getting started

The internet has been a game changer for the transgender community. Before this many people experiencing gender dysphoria did not even have the words for how they were feeling, never mind the information and support of the online community. For many, this was an incredibly isolating experience.

I remember being at a conference once where the room was filled with baby boomer generation transgender women. The speaker asked the audience how many had felt growing up, that they were the only one on the planet to feel this way. Almost every hand in the room shot up.

Unfortunately, however, the quality of information online is variable. There are few fields in medicine that have as much myth and in some cases misinformation. Also, much of the information can be difficult for the average patient to read and understand. Having said that my gender affirmation surgery patients tend to be most well-informed patients I have.

First steps

Many towns and cities have local support groups, which can be extremely helpful for patients and their families even if just virtual. Here many patients will begin to find their transgender community.

Using online resources, the next step for many will be to reach out to a savvy provider.

Mental Health Professionals

An early step for many in exploring their gender identity further and if appropriate, transitioning will be to find a mental health professional who has experience in this area. Most patients will find their mental health professional online often through "word of mouth", on social media or from the recommendation of other patients. Although this can be really tough for somebody living in a rural area many professionals can now do "virtual consults" to save on travel.

Counseling can be expensive with limited insurance coverage. Some mental health professionals can offer a sliding scale to help low income patients.

Mental health professionals can offer transgender and gender non-conforming individuals a range of very important services apart from just helping explore gender identity. They can help with the process of coming out and help support friends and family members through a patient's transition. They can also provide information to patients with regard to gender expression and medical interventions. They can help manage coexisting mental health issues such as anxiety or depression. Where appropriate they can assess and refer for hormone and surgical treatments. They will write the all-important "WPATH letter". Sometimes a second mental health letter is needed, and they may be able to refer to a colleague for that evaluation also.

Primary Care Doctors

Some lucky patients may be able to find a primary care doctor who has experience in treating transgender and gender non-conforming patients.

This doc may be able to prescribe hormones or refer to another physician who does. In the future, it's expected that this will be within the scope of practice of all primary care docs considering how common being transgender is.

What is "WPATH"?

Early on in a patient's care they may hear terms like "WPATH letter" or "WPATH standards of care". Obviously, many folks won't know what this means.

WPATH stands for the "World Professional Association of Transgender Health". It is a large professional organization of multiple types of providers (mental health professionals, doctors, nurses) that take part in caring for patients of all gender identities. It is an international organization that promotes education, research and advocacy in transgender health.

Standards of Care

One of the most important things WPATH does is produce the "Standards of Care."

This is a document, which outlines best-practice guidelines for taking care of patients with gender dysphoria.

It is an easy read (120 pages) for doctors and patients alike and available in many languages on their website www.WPATH.org.

Version 7 of this document was published in 2011 and at the time of writing this version 8 is in the works.

Gatekeeping?

Some of the most important things in this document are the recommendations on requirements that should be met by a patient before undergoing a treatment.

The goal of these recommendations is "harm reduction". They are designed as check points to make sure that this is the right treatment for that patient and, most importantly, the right time to undergo a procedure.

Different surgeries have different requirements. For example, genital surgeries have the most detailed requirements. Patients have to have 2 mental health referrals as well as a minimum of a year on hormones and a year of "real life experience" in their gender role.

They also require that the patient be otherwise well enough mentally and physically to undergo surgery. Doing surgery at the wrong time can be devastating. If the patient is not physically fit for a big procedure like this, it can be life threatening. Many of the surgeries require a lot of work on the patient's part to take care of their new anatomy. If a patient is, say, too depressed for example to do the post-op care bad complications can happen.

While a lot of doctors may sometimes vary slightly from these guidelines to make sure the individual patient has the best possible care, most doctors will broadly stick to these guidelines.

Insurance Company Policies

In addition, many insurance companies who now provide coverage for these treatments will also want to see that the WPATH requirements have been met.

At the time of writing this WPATH version eight is being written. We may see a move towards a more "informed consent" model where there is less emphasis on referrals and letters "clearing" a patient and more of an emphasis on the patient fully understanding their choices and having bodily autonomy.

WPATH letters can be a pain to gather for patients and providers alike however most providers agree that for such life changing surgeries it's good to have experts involved to make sure it's the right time.

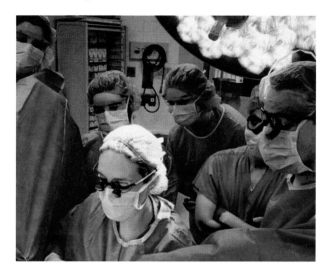

Figure 3 Dr Gallagher and her team perform vaginoplasty.

Finding a Surgeon

Many different types of surgeons can be involved in gender affirmation surgery as it is at the intersection of different fields. Plastic surgeons represent the majority, but there are also gynecologists, urologists and ENT surgeons to name a few.

The internet and social media are usually the biggest source of information for patients as many previous patients are willing to share their experiences and results.

Some things to keep in mind when considering surgeons.

1. Is your surgeon board certified?

In the United States this is one of the most important check-points we have when evaluating a surgeon's credentials. For example, in order to be certified by the American Board of Plastic Surgery a doctor has to go through many years of intense training after medical school, gain certain experience and standards as well as pass rigorous examinations. This is a very fair question for a perspective surgeon therefore – are you board certified and in what field? It is important to know not all boards are created equally. There are a number of agencies out there that offer "board certification" to a doctor without much training or certification involved!

Your surgeon should be certified by a board that is recognized by the American Board of Medical Specialties. You can check if your surgeon is certified on their website www.abms.org .

2. Can you see before and after pictures?

Again, this is a fair request – maybe your surgeon is a good safe surgeon, but do you like their particular results? Aesthetics are very important in many gender affirmation procedures.

3. Do you "click" with that surgeon? Can you understand what they are communicating to you about the surgery?

A lot of explaining and teaching often needs to be done so patients can properly take care of themselves after the procedure and learn to use their new anatomy. It's important that your surgeon and their team can get this across to you. If you can't understand them before surgery, it's probably going to be just as difficult or worse after surgery.

Surgery Overseas

Traditionally many patients had no option but to seek treatment is other countries. South East Asia offered patients affordable care often without the long waitlists of the United States.

There is no doubt that there are extremely experienced expert surgeons in other countries, and I have certainly trained with some of them.

There are however 2 major concerns about surgery abroad.

Is it Safe?

Firstly, medical care in the United States, while it is expensive, is without a doubt world class. While the surgeon abroad may indeed be technically excellent complications can happen with surgery. For example, if the patient were to suffer a heart attack, they would have to make do with the standards of care in that country. This can be a very scary predicament to be in. In other countries sometimes the same checks and balances we have here in the US just don't apply. With language barriers it can be impossible for patients to fully understand what's going on. I have taken care of some unfortunate patients who have returned home after a procedure abroad with horrible complications that would be rare in the US.

What happens afterwards?

Secondly, we always have to remember what happens after surgery? Many patients will travel far distances even in their home country to get care. Its important to ask what systems the surgeon and their team have in place to answer questions or maybe communicate with other doctors back home.

For these reasons and the fact that there are now many more options closer to home I would not want my loved one travelling for surgery out of the country. You only get one body; you must be careful with it!

How to make Surgery Happen

Timing

By the time a patient is considering gender affirmation surgery, usually they are anxious to move along with their transition. However, it is so important to make sure it is the correct time to embark on surgeries. Some surgeries even without complications take months to recover from and a patient needs to make sure they have all the social, physical, emotional and financial resources to follow through and look after their new anatomy.

Insurance Financial Considerations

Transitioning is very expensive business!

Funding your own Surgery

Prices of surgery vary widely, depending on the complexity of the case.

Travel for the patient and their companion should be factored in as well as arrangements for missing work.

A "cushion" of extra funds is strongly recommended before proceeding with the surgery. If a patient, for whatever reason needs and unexpected repeat surgery to treat a problem many surgeons wont charge for their time, however the patient will need to pay for the anesthesia and operating room costs.

There also can be other hidden expenses such as dressings, medications and transport to take into consideration.

Insurance

Certain states in the USA have laws in place which protect the transgender patient and allow them to undergo the medically necessary procedures for treatment of gender dysphoria.

For all the other states, as a general rule Medicaid plans will not cover surgeries but sometimes Medicare will.

All employees of agencies with Federal funding have access to benefits that cover procedures.

In the case of private insurance, it usually depends on whether or not the patient's employer chooses benefits to cover procedures to treat gender dysphoria.

It can be often very difficult to figure out whether you are covered or not and what exact requirements are needed before surgery according to the policy.

If a patient is covered, the policy must be examined to see what criteria must be met. Whereas previously providers were regarded as the "gatekeepers" we could say the new gate keepers are often the policy writers!

Usually these requirements will be based on the WPATH Standards of Care but not always. A cynic could conclude that these sometimes-bizarre requirements are designed to make access to surgery as difficult as possible.

Another problem is the fact that an insurance policy may cover some codes (creation of the vagina) but not others (creation of the clitoris) that are a routine part of the surgery.

For these reasons working with insurance can be notoriously difficult.

When all the necessary documentation is gathered and once the patient is ready to undergo surgery, the surgeon's office will submit a letter to the insurance company seeking permission to proceed with the gender affirmation surgery with all this relevant documentation and usually photos. Once the insurance company authorizes the procedure usually a date is set with the surgeon.

The time it takes for an insurance company to respond is highly variable and can take in some cases 12 weeks, so it is important to plan ahead!

The busiest time for all surgeons is usually December – this is because insurance deductibles will have been met so patients clamor to get their procedures in before the end of the year.

Holidays and school breaks are very busy also usually.

Age and gender affirmation surgery

Is there an upper or lower age limit for surgery?

We do not necessarily have a "cut-off" age for surgeries.

In my career I have operated on transitioning patients as young as 16 and as old as 72.

We believe in individualized care for our patients and carefully weigh up the risks and benefits of gender affirming surgery for each patient.

Mature Patients

Some gender affirmation procedures are minor while some are major. With age the risks of complications do increase but in a healthy individual, even the most invasive procedures may be possible.

In general, your surgeon will estimate your risks by reviewing your full medical history and performing a physical. For the more invasive procedures such as vaginoplasty we will order additional tests or may have a cardiologist or anesthesiologist also see you.

It is worth remembering that there are less invasive options available for mature patients also for example a patient may opt not to undergo a full vaginoplasty and instead undergo an orchiectomy and scrotoplasty or a zero-depth procedure.

Younger Patients

The World Professional Association of Transgender Health publishes standards of care recommending that surgery not be undertaken until the patient is of the age of consent, therefore 18 in the USA.

However, we prefer to individualize patient's care and recognize that certain patients may be mature enough to make these decisions and indeed may hugely benefit from gender affirmation long before their 18th birthday.

This may be particularly true in the case of top surgery. A teenager may be much better served undergoing a surgery during their summer vacation from high school with the support of parents rather than trying to recover in a college dorm.

Working with our mental health professionals is also very important in the case of the younger patient in order to assess the maturity of the patient in making this life-altering decision and readiness for postoperative care.

Mental Health and Transitioning

By Vanessa de la Llama, MS, LMHC

Hello, my name is Vanessa de la Llama, I am a Licensed Mental Health Counselor, and I specialize in working with Trans clients. With so many paths and options to take in our world today, it is incredibly important to know and understand your options and paths for your treatment. Working through an issue is already hard to begin with but having the correct tools and information at hand makes this process smoother. No matter where you are in your transition journey, please know that information is always power. Know your rights, know your options and know your providers. As a Licensed Mental Health Counselor, my job is not only to help process emotions and feelings, my job is also to educate and to help my clients find the right fit for them whether it be therapy, hormone treatment, cosmetic surgery or procedures, and transition surgery. My job is to help guide, weigh pros and cons, as well as work with the clients through every stage.

So first things first, you need to find a mental health professional, whether it be a psychiatrist, psychologist, Licensed Mental Health Counselor or Licensed Clinical Social Worker, here is where you want to start. Whether you have spoken to family or friends about your feelings and emotions, it is always good to start with a professional. Like I said, knowledge is power, so the more educated we are about a topic, the better off we are at making decisions and understanding what it is that we truly want and need.

How do you find a mental health professional? If you are a minor, talk with a parent or guardian to help you find a provider through either your insurance or outside your insurance network. If you are over 18, then either check who is covered by your insurance or do some research and find providers that specialize in Trans clients. These providers can be found through directories such as WPATH (World Professional Association for Transgender Health) and NQTTCN (National Queer and Trans Therapists of Color Network). These national organizations have directories dedicated to providers who specialize in working with Trans clients and is a good source to go through due to the fact that the therapist you find should have a solid background on these organizations' ethical practices. Therapy is therapy, but there are providers who are more specialized in this area than others. Good screening questions when choosing your therapist should always be if they are part of any organizations or if they have had any specialized trainings such as Transgender Care Trainings or other certifications. This will ensure that you are partnering up with a provider who is as ready as possible to help you with your specific needs.

A good solid therapeutic relationship is vital. Picture this, every human has their likes and dislikes. So when you go walking down the aisles of your nearest convenience store, you often choose a product you have tried time and time again and that has been successful for you. Now it is not to say that the products you pass on are bad, they just do not mix well with your genetic code, complexion, etc. I like to compare therapist shopping to product shopping. All therapists offer great benefits and are all trained to help with mental health issues, but depending on your personality and

issues, a specific therapist may not be right for you. As a female cisgender, I love a great facial product, but finding one that works for my skin without breaking out is another issue all in itself. This is why it is crucial that you either have a quick 20-minute consultation with your therapist before your first session or screen them appropriately when scheduling an appointment. Test try them. Once again, knowledge is key, so use the internet and referrals to find your best fit. Through my experience, most clients have seen 2-3 therapists before settling in with one. This is someone you are trusting with all your intimate information and details; it is worth searching for your best match.

Before continuing on to the next steps, I would like to bring up insurance. Giant elephant in the room. We all have different insurances and each one of our plans cover different options, so it is very important to take a look at finances while going through this journey. Not everyone is so blessed as to be able to pay for medical expenses out of pocket. I am aware of how finances play a huge role in everyone's life, and how much control it can hold. This is why it is critical to look at your healthcare benefits and what your possibility of paying out of pocket will look like. This is not to deter you from reaching out and getting services, absolutely not, but like I said, knowledge is power, and knowing how to manage your money and insurance provider during this process is important. Insurances cover therapy, medication management, hormone therapy (with proper diagnosis), and even parts of gender affirmations procedures and surgeries (with proper diagnoses and letters). My personal and professional recommendation is that you or your guardian call the insurance company and ask every question regarding:

- what is needed for services to be covered (referrals, letters, diagnoses, etc.)

- what specific services are covered under your plan?

- how to get reimbursed for out-of-network services?

- how much of those services are covered?

- what referrals and fees will be involved?

I am a big fan of making sure my insurance provider does their job to tell me everything I need to know in a language that I can understand. This can and probably will be a tedious process, just know it is for the client's best interest and benefit.

So, you found your perfect therapist? Fantastic! Now we are moving onto what to expect during your first session. First sessions are always heavy information based such as limits of confidentiality, rights of the patient/client, demographics, personal vocabulary (i.e. verbiage), and history. It is a lot of information bringing on the patients/client's side. This sounds exhausting, I know, but the foremost expert on the client is the client, so understanding and listening to the client's truth and understanding is most important to a therapist. Depending on your therapist and if you are working through insurances, initial sessions last anywhere from 45 minutes to 110 minutes. If you are going through insurance, your session length and amount will be limited. Going out of network gives you more flexibility, although it is the more expensive option. If you have access, make sure to bring all your past mental health history documents and files to your first session. This helps the therapist have a clearer understanding of your medical history, as well as giving the therapist a more concrete understanding of the issue in a handwritten document by another medical professional. Not only does this add knowledge, but also adds proof and trailing's that help establish that the client has been suffering with mental health issues and is in current need of help.

Moving right along to your second therapy session. The therapy process has no time frame, no date frame, no expectations. The reason I bring this up is because I constantly get questions from parents and clients asking me how long they will be in therapy for, how long it will take to get a letter, and how long will it take the client to get better. First things first, time is irrelevant here. Yes, there will be a time and place when both the therapist and client believe the client is ready for the proceeding steps, yes there will be improvement, and yes, there will be hope and a light at the end of the tunnel but this cannot be rushed. Every person has a different story and every person will react differently to therapy this is an ongoing process. Moving forward to getting hormone treatment or surgeries will not take years, it is all

part of the process. Having a healthy and open relationship with your therapist is crucial in this step.

Therapy will consist of a mix of individual therapy, family therapy and couples' therapy. The reason for this is that transition effects everyone surrounding the client, and to ensure that the client has a heathy and safe environment to grow and develop, it is key to have all major players in a client's life involved appropriately. Each type of therapy will come with due time, and that all depends on how ready and prepared the client is to share their journey with others. As a client you should never be pushed, harassed or tricked into anything other than individual therapy. During your therapy process, these big decisions will be discussed and chosen together. Remember that 'family' and 'parents' do not have to be biological. People most important to the client should be involved in their transition journey.

Please note that therapy is not limited to emotions. Depending on where you are in your transition, you might be already completing procedures or hormone therapy, all this should be discussed with your therapist. It is valuable for your medical providers to know what is happening in all stages of your transition, and that all providers are on the same page as you the client. This makes your transition providers much more fluid and allows for proper and vital communication between providers. Make sure you have your providers sign a Release of Information form so that your providers legally have the right to discuss your case with one another.

Referral and recommendation letters.

Depending on where you are in your transition, you might want to start hormone therapy or have some surgeries or procedures completed. I am not a gatekeeper. I am not the troll who holds your future in their hands. Please do not look at your therapist as a gatekeeper, we are not here to hold a letter in front of you and dangle it until we hear what we want. As mentioned before, all steps in transition come in their time, and so will your letters. Therapists and other mental health professionals trained to work with the trans community should be knowledgeable about child and human development and will work with the client, family and other health providers to ensure the client is

receiving the appropriate services at the best time possible. Another good way to screen your therapist is to ask them how long it would take for them to get a medical letter. If the therapist has a time frame or charges you specifically for the letter, I don't think they would be your best choice. Your health professionals should be looking out for your best interests, always.

Diagnoses and therapeutic interventions.

For those of you who are already with a health professional, you might have noticed that you were diagnosed with Gender Dysphoria (F64.2 or F64.1). It is key for Trans clients to understand where the diagnosis comes from and how it is they fit into it. Now most clients will have a mixture of PTSD, or Anxiety, or Depression with Gender Dysphoria. This is what we call in the mental health world comorbidity. There is a plethora of comorbidity options; make sure to have your provider teach and educate you on these diagnoses and verbiage. This will help you be more 'eye to eye' with your provider. Your therapist or provider can help translate any medical language that you may not understand. Below is criteria mental health professionals use to diagnose Gender Dysphoria.

The *Diagnostic and Statistical Manual of Mental Disorders* (DSM-5) provides for one overarching diagnosis of gender dysphoria with separate specific criteria for children and for adolescents and adults.

- In adolescents and adults gender dysphoria diagnosis involves a difference between one's experienced/expressed gender and assigned gender, and significant distress or problems functioning. It lasts at least six months and is shown by at least two of the following:

  1. A marked incongruence between one's experienced/expressed gender and primary and/or secondary sex characteristics

  2. A strong desire to be rid of one's primary and/or secondary sex characteristics

  3. A strong desire for the primary and/or secondary sex characteristics of the other gender

  4. A strong desire to be of the other gender

  5. A strong desire to be treated as the other gender

  6. A strong conviction that one has the typical feelings and reactions of the other gender

- In children, gender dysphoria diagnosis involves at least six of the following and an associated significant distress or impairment in function, lasting at least six months.

  1. A strong desire to be of the other gender or an insistence that one is the other gender

  2. A strong preference for wearing clothes typical of the opposite gender

  3. A strong preference for cross-gender roles in make-believe play or fantasy play

  4. A strong preference for the toys, games or activities stereotypically used or engaged in by the other gender

  5. A strong preference for playmates of the other gender

  6. A strong rejection of toys, games and activities typical of one's assigned gender

  7. A strong dislike of one's sexual anatomy

8. A strong desire for the physical sex characteristics that match one's experienced gender

For children, cross-gender behaviors may start between ages 2 and 4, the same age at which most typically developing children begin showing gendered behaviors and interests. Gender atypical behavior is common among young children and may be part of normal development. Children who meet the criteria for gender dysphoria may or may not continue to experience it into adolescence and adulthood. Some research shows that children who had more intense symptoms and distress, who were more persistent, insistent and consistent in their cross-gender statements and behaviors, and who used more declarative statements ("I am a boy (or girl)" rather than "I want to be a boy (or girl)") were more likely to become transgender adults.

Basic definitions/verbiage to know (American Psychiatric Association, 2020):

- Gender - denotes the public (and usually legally recognized) lived role as boy or girl, man or woman. Biological factors combined with social and psychological factors contribute to gender development.

- Assigned gender - refers to a person's initial assignment as male or female at birth. It is based on the child's genitalia and other visible physical sex characteristics.

- Gender-atypical - refers to physical features or behaviors that are not typical of individuals of the same assigned gender in a given society.

- Gender-nonconforming - refers to behaviors that are not typical of individuals with the same assigned gender in a given society.

- Gender reassignment - denotes an official (and usually legal) change of gender.

- Gender identity - is a category of social identity and refers to an individual's identification as male, female or, occasionally, some category other than male or female. It is one's deeply held core sense of being male, female, some of both or neither, and does not always correspond to biological sex.

- Gender dysphoria - as a general descriptive term refers to an individual's discontent with the assigned gender. It is more specifically defined when used as a diagnosis.

- Transgender - refers to the broad spectrum of individuals who transiently or persistently identify with a gender different from their gender at birth. (Note: the term transgendered is not generally used.)

- Transsexual - refers to an individual who seeks, or has undergone, a social transition from male to female or female to male. In many, but not all, cases this also involves a physical transition through cross-sex hormone treatment and genital surgery (sex reassignment surgery).

- Genderqueer - blurring the lines around gender identity and sexual orientation. Genderqueer individuals typically embrace a fluidity of gender identity and sometimes sexual orientation.

- Gender fluidity - having different gender identities at different times.

- Agendered - 'without gender,' individuals identifying as having no gender identity.

- Cisgender - describes individuals whose gender identity or expression aligns with the sex assigned to them at birth.

- Gender expansiveness - conveys a wider, more flexible range of gender identity and/or expression than typically associated with the binary gender system.

- Gender expression - the manner in which a person communicates about gender to others through external means such as clothing, appearance, or mannerisms. This communication may be conscious or subconscious and may or may not reflect their gender identity or sexual orientation.

There are many organizations and associations throughout the United States that help Transgendered youth and adults with support. National organizations such as The *National* Center for *Transgender* Equality, GLAAD, *National Transgender* Advocacy Coalition, Gender Proud, and Trans Latina Coalition all have seminars, lectures, online trainings and videos to help families and friends find support in the world. Having support groups and friends in these organizations help clients find real world support from others in their same exact predicament. This is always a plus and a benefit to have on a daily basis. I have sent countless clients and parents to these seminars, and I often find myself scoping through my local associations to see what events they have in my area.

Therapy is not to frighten you. I often hear from clients that they were more hesitant to speak to a therapist than any other step in their transition. And my only response to that is to thank them for taking the leap of faith. Transitioning is a terrifying yet liberating process. As a cisgender woman and therapist, I cannot even begin to fathom the depth and strength it takes for a client to go through this process. My job is not to fathom, it is to help you through this process, with a guide and support in hand for every step. Wherever you are in your transition journey, please know that you are not alone and that you have an endless amount of support and information to help through this time. Please always reach out to your mental health professional with any issues or concerns.

Fertility Preservation

By Amelia McLennan, MD

What is fertility preservation?

Fertility preservation refers to the process of collecting and freezing eggs, sperm, and/or embryos that can be used for future childbearing. There are many reasons why people choose to undergo these procedures, but in the case of transgender and non-binary individuals hormones and surgery can make it difficult or impossible to have biological children without undergoing this.

How does it work?

The process is different depending on whether the goal is to save/freeze oocytes (eggs), sperm, or embryos (eggs that have been fertilized with sperm in the lab).

Sperm freezing (or cryopreservation) is the most straightforward. After consultation at a cryopreservation facility ("sperm bank") or fertility clinic, a sample is produced via masturbation/ejaculation, usually at the storage facility, and the facility tests the sample for quality and infection, then stores it in a specialized freezer until you are ready to use it. Usually it is recommended to store multiple samples to ensure there is enough for multiple attempts at pregnancy if needed. There is typically a one-time cost for collecting, testing and freezing the sample, (usually a few hundred dollars), and then an annual cost for storage.

Oocyte cryopreservation (egg freezing), is a bit more complicated. Essentially, you must undergo the first half of an in-vitro fertilization (IVF) cycle. The process is done under the care of a reproductive endocrinologist (an OB/GYN specializing in fertility treatments) and typically takes about 1-2 months. First, the menstrual cycle may need to be regulated using combined oral contraceptives (birth control pills containing estrogen and progesterone). Then the ovaries are stimulated using a variety of hormonal medications (by mouth and/or by injection) to produce many more eggs than they would during a typical monthly cycle. Once the eggs are mature, you undergo a minor surgical procedure under light anesthesia to collect the eggs (this is done using a needle guided by ultrasound through the wall of the vagina into the ovary). Depending on your age and other factors, you may produce anywhere from zero to 20 or more mature eggs from one cycle. It is sometimes recommended to undergo multiple cycles to ensure that there are enough eggs to produce a normal pregnancy, as each egg only has a small chance of surviving the entire process of creating a baby (defrosting, fertilization with sperm, growing enough to be implanted, being genetically normal, and making it through pregnancy). It may take 20 or more frozen eggs to have one healthy baby. The cost of an IVF cycle varies, and may be partially or completely covered by insurance, but the out-of-pocket cost can be about $10,000-$20,000 if not covered. In addition, there is an annual fee to store frozen eggs in a specialized freezer at a fertility clinic.

Embryo cryopreservation involves going through the egg collection process as described above, but before freezing the eggs are fertilized with sperm and grown in the lab for a few days to create embryos.

The benefit of embryo freezing is that frozen embryos have a higher pregnancy success rate than frozen eggs, and there is the option of doing genetic testing on the embryos before freezing so that you are able to only store ones that you know are genetically normal and likely to produce a healthy pregnancy/baby. In order to create embryos, you must have sperm available at the time of egg collection, either from a known donor/partner or an anonymous sperm donor.

What are the risks?

Sperm freezing has essentially no risks.

Going through the process of ovarian stimulation and egg collection has some risks. The various hormonal medications used commonly have some side effects (these vary from person to person but can include nausea/vomiting, bloating, headaches, pain at injection site, mood swings, and others). There is also a small risk of a serious complication called ovarian hyperstimulation syndrome, where the ovaries get very enlarged and may leak fluid into the abdomen, leading to severe pain and frequently hospitalization. Fertility specialists take every precaution to avoid this complication and treat it promptly if it occurs. The egg retrieval process is associated with some discomfort during your recovery and may require a few days off work. There is a small risk of serious complications such as heavy bleeding or injury to nearby structures such as bladder and bowel. Overall this is a very safe procedure with minimal risk.

All fertility preservation procedures carry the risk of not being successful in creating pregnancies in the future.

How do I use my frozen eggs/sperm/embryos?

Once you are ready to start a family, preserved eggs/sperm/embryos

can be used to attempt pregnancy, either for you or your partner (if one of you has a uterus) or in a gestational carrier/surrogate.

Frozen sperm can be used either for insemination (where sperm is inserted either in the vagina or the uterus at the time of natural ovulation to hopefully allow fertilization to happen "naturally"), or to fertilize previously frozen or fresh eggs as part of in-vitro fertilization (IVF).

Frozen eggs must be fertilized in the lab with sperm (from a partner, known or anonymous donor) to create embryos which then can be transferred to anyone who has a uterus to carry a pregnancy.

More resources:

American Association of Tissue Banks (AATB)
American Society for Reproductive Medicine (ASRM)
Livestrong Fertility
Resolve
Society for Assisted Reproductive Technology (SART)

Section 1

Healthcare for Transfeminine Patients and Non-Binary Assigned Male at Birth Patients

1. Feminizing Hormones

By Sidhbh Gallagher

There are few areas in medicine with so much mystery and controversy as feminizing hormones.

Many doctors have different preferences on the safest and most effective medicines. Traditionally each hormone prescriber would often use their own unique cocktail. Understandably, therefore, this can be really confusing for patients.

As more research comes to light on this topic hopefully, we will see this as a thing of the past and the professional societies are working on guidelines to help standardize treatments.

When are hormones right?

Up until a few years ago it was recommended that a patient always have a letter confirming a diagnosis of gender dysphoria from a mental health professional before starting hormone therapy. There has, however, been a trend towards an "informed consent" model whereby the patient's right to make choices for their own body is recognized and as long as the patient is fully informed of the risks, they may start hormone therapy. As long as the hormone prescriber is comfortable making the diagnosis of gender dysphoria, they will use this model. Studies have shown that regret is very rare even with the informed consent model. Before any medical treatment the provider must of course make sure the patient is fit and healthy enough to undergo treatment and that there are no health issues that make it riskier.

What drugs will I take?

Two drugs are usually needed in order to feminize.

Firstly, estrogen is the mainstay of treatment for transgender women but in addition she will need something to block the powerful effects of testosterone (unless the testicles have already been removed).

Hormones

Modern estrogen (estradiol) formulations have lower risks than the types used in the past. Most patients will take this in the form of pills once or twice a day.

Progestins (the other female sex hormone) can also be used but come with a potential risk of breast cancer, mood swings and blood clots. The benefits of progestins are less clear. Theoretically, as this hormone plays a role in breast development it may help in breast feminization, however this is controversial and has never been proven. Therefore, not all prescribers will use this hormone.

Blockers

There are a few different options for blocking testosterone. The most common is spironolactone. This is in fact a water pill (diuretic), which also blocks testosterone.

Blood tests need to be monitored as in some patients spironolactone can raise potassium, which could be dangerous.

Other options are finasteride (in most patients this is not as effective).

Leuprolide is another option which is in a family of drugs known as GNRH analogues- these however tend to be quite pricey.

What are the dangers/ side effects?

Many would agree that the medical community has been quite behind in figuring out what the real risks of hormones in transgender women actually are. Most of our current beliefs come from the studies where only post-menopausal, non-transgender women were enrolled. Also, much of the data comes from studies using older formulations of estrogen so this information really doesn't translate well to the transgender population.

Side effects of estrogens

Annoying symptoms some patients may have on estrogens include migraines, mood swings, hot flashes, and weight gain. Also, some patients will experience a drop in libido and most will experience loss of erections. If a transgender woman would prefer to still be able to have erections her hormone provider can prescribe medications like Viagra to help. It is very unpredictable which if any unwanted side effects a patient may have as many different factors play into a patient's response to hormones including genetics.

Dangers of Estrogens

The biggest fear physicians have about starting estrogens in any patient is the increased risk of blood clots. Blood clots (which often form in the legs) can actually be lethal if they travel to the lungs and cause a pulmonary embolism.

The good news is that the risk in another-wise healthy patient seems to still be very low when the modern formulations of estrogen are used. In addition, patches can be used if the patient has additional risk factors. When a patient is over 40 many doctors will recommend using a patch. Smoking is a risk factor for blood clots so therefore it is strongly encouraged that smoking should be stopped prior to starting estrogen therapy.

Fact: Hormones taken by mouth have a higher risk of causing blood clots.

In patients who have had blood clots in the past or are at increased risk the hormone provider will assess the risks of estrogen on an individual basis.

Other rarer potential risks of estrogen include autoimmune diseases and pituitary tumors. There are only a few cases reported due to estrogens that we know of.

Side effects of Spironolactone

As previously mentioned, spironolactone is a water pill or diuretic. Patients may notice increased thirst and urination when they start on it initially. Also, some patients may notice they get lightheaded when standing up quickly. These symptoms all tend to pass.

Dangers of Spironolactone

Patients who have kidney disease or are taking other certain types of medications may not be able to take spironolactone. This is because spironolactone increases levels of potassium in the blood. At high levels potassium can be extremely dangerous causing heart rhythm problems among other dangers. This is why your doctor will want to monitor blood tests to check potassium after starting spironolactone.

Fact: a common side effect of spironolactone is dizziness, especially when the patient stands up

What checks do I need?

Hormones and blockers are powerful drugs that can really do wonders physically and emotionally – they can however potentially cause harm so your hormone provider will keep a close eye especially at first when starting. This is to make sure they are working adequately and that they aren't causing harm.

Doctors will usually monitor for feminizing and adverse effects every 3 months for the first year, then every 6–12 months. A recent study showed that it takes an average of 9 months for hormone levels to reach a steady state, so patience is needed.

Your doctor will obtain baseline blood tests to see where you are starting from (hematocrit, prolactin and lipid profile) and monitor at follow-up visits.

In addition, they will monitor serum testosterone during the first 6 months until levels drop to <55 ng/dL and monitor serum estradiol (estrogen levels) at follow-up visits; target 100–200 pg/mL.

In addition, changes in sex hormones may affect bone density so they often will check this if a patient is at risk for osteoporosis.

What changes can I expect to see?

Hormone effects are slow and gradual often taking 18 – 24 months to fully kick in.

- Breast growth,
- Increased body fat,
- Slowed growth of body and facial hair,
- Decreased testicular size and

- Decreased erectile function.
- Changes in libido
- Reduced or absent sperm count and ejaculatory fluid

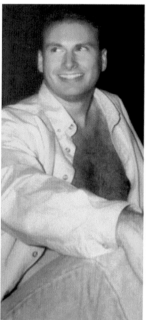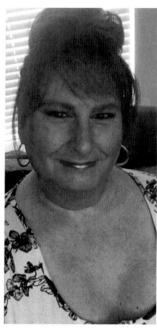

Figure 4 Adrienne's transformation.

What about feminizing hormones in youth?

Transgender youth require a multidisciplinary specialized team.

Hormone blockers have been used to stop the development of secondary sexual characteristics – which can be associated with severe dysphoria. The endocrine society generally recommends starting estrogen aged 16. However, this is usually done on an individualized basis, depending on how long the youth has been on blockers. If a patient has been on blockers for a long time with no sex hormones this can lead to problems with low bone mineral density.

What about feminizing hormones in old age?

There is not a lot known, unfortunately, about feminizing hormones in more mature patients. There have certainly been reports of patients starting and doing well on cross-hormonal therapy at more advanced ages. Older patients tend to have more medical problems so it stands to reason that starting hormones may be riskier. Each patient can decide this on an individual bases along with their doctor.

Considering that in the US the average age of menopause is 50 – patients will sometimes stop estrogen around that age. If the patient hasn't undergone orchiectomy, she may indeed experience masculinizing effects.

What happens hormones after bottom surgery?

Once the testicles are removed a transgender woman will no longer require a testosterone blocker. Also, in most the estrogen dose needed will drop by 25%-50%.

Fertility and Transitioning

Before beginning hormones, it is important for patients to consider whether having biological children is important to them. Once hormones have been started the quantity and quality of sperm produced decreases and often stops. This however is unpredictable and therefore contraception is still necessary to avoid unwanted pregnancies.

Freezing sperm or "cryopreservation" is the best option for patients who may want to have genetically related children in the future. Unfortunately, often this is not covered by insurance. There is usually a yearly storage fee also to keep the sperm.

Patients can try to do this after being on hormones. It is variable how well sperm production will return however after being on hormones, so it is best to consider this early in transition.

The future may bring more fertility options for transgender women.

For example, more than 42 uterine transplants have been carried out around the world in non-transgender women and at least twelve live births have been reported. An interesting study from London suggested that this may well be an option

1.

for transgender women – with the donation of a uterus and a vagina. In this way transgender women may be able to in fact experience pregnancy someday. This technology is however still very early and not at all widely available.

2. Non-operative Facial Feminization and Skin care

Dr. Sidhbh Gallagher

Non-Operative Facial Feminization

Injectables such as Botox and fillers have been game changers in the world of aesthetics and anti-aging. These options are usually more affordable and appealing to patients who wish to improve their features without undergoing the knife.

These techniques, however, can also be used to help feminize the face. While obviously not as effective as surgery some cleverly placed filler or Botox can be very affirming in patients who are either not ready to undergo surgery or don't have access to it.

In this chapter we will discuss what treatments can be used either to start a patient on her facial feminization journey or to help with it.

- Hair removal
- Fillers
- Botox
- Lasers, Peels and Mechanical Abrasion
- Skin care for the transfeminine patient

Injectables

Using fillers to reverse the signs of aging can have a feminizing effect. As we age, we lose volume from our cheeks. The inner cheek is the first place to loose volume around the mid to late thirties. Replacing this volume improves the shape of the cheeks as well as often helping to decrease lines and bags.

The lips can be enhanced very effectively with lip injections to pump out and enlarge the vermillion (red) part of the lip.

Botulinum Toxin

What is Botulinum Toxin?

Botox is a brand name of one of the most popular types of Botulinum Toxin on the market. This is a toxin which, if injected in small safe doses it was found would stop facial muscles from moving as much.

A big reason we form lines on the face is because of the constant pulling of the muscles of facial expression. It was found if that movement is decreased the lines also soften and indeed if kept up may not form.

The first place it was applied commonly was the forehead and to get rid of the "11 lines" or frown lines between the eyebrows. Since then Botox has been used for countless other beauty reasons beyond just this. Indeed, an advanced Botox injector will be able to evaluate a patient's face and inject catering just to that particular patient. Every face is somewhat asymmetrical, and the muscles may be more active on one side of the face compared to the other. It is worth seeing a very well-trained injector such as a plastic surgeon as they know the anatomy better and will use an individualized approach to identify and treat the exact areas causing the lines. Though on the surface this may seem more expensive, its often the case that you will get a lot more "bang for your buck" than a cookie-cutter approach. Botox is usually charged by the unit and every patient will require or want a different amount – most starting doses are 30-100 units.

Anti-aging Effects

In most cases transgender women over the age of 35 could benefit from some of the usual antiaging applications of Botox to help "soften" their features. This can include lines on the forehead, 11 lines between the eyes, crow's feet at the corners of the eyes, "bunny lines" at the bridge of the nose and vertical lines around the mouth. Also, Botox can be used to relax a dimpled chin.

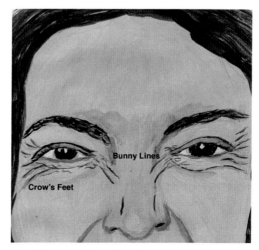

Figure 5 Lines that form around eyes that are treatable with Botox.

How to tell if Botox will benefit you?

The best time to start treating lines on the face is when they are just becoming "static lines". What does this mean? There are 2 types of lines- dynamic lines are the lines that go away when we relax (which even babies have when they scrunch up their faces). These eventually may become static lines – meaning we can still see that line even when the face is completely at rest.

They will be faint at first. If we start consistently using Botox at the age they first appear, those lines should disappear and hopefully will never even develop.

In the case of older patients with static lines, there is only so much Botox can do. Often times however, Botox can help at least soften these lines. If your surgeon points you in the direction of another treatment such as surgery, however, Botox likely may be a waste of your money.

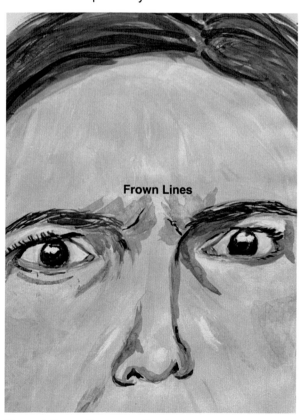

Figure 6 Frown lines are effectively softened with Botox.

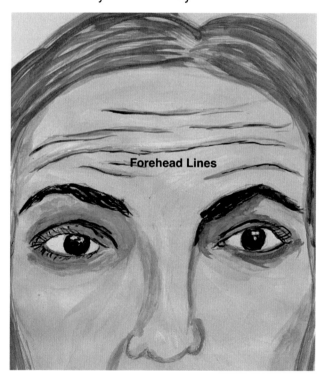

Figure 7 Forehead lines can effectively be treated with Botox.

Most Caucasian patients are beginning to develop these at the age of 35 (other races usually later).

Botox can however be used in other ways in some cases to help feminize the face.

Jaw Contouring

Botox can, in some cases help soften the appearance of a "square jaw". In patients the angle of the jaw, which, in men can have that square appearance is made up of not only the jawbone but the masseter muscle also. Botox shots (usually about 3 a side) can be used to shrink this muscle down and therefore give a more feminine, oval shape to the face. Botox effects are unfortunately temporary, but many patients will have results lasting up to 6 months.

The masseter is also usually responsible for patients who grind their teeth so weakening that muscle can help get rid of that problem also.

This must be done by an experienced injector as injecting Botox on the lower face can cause problems if it gets into the wrong muscles. The most common side effect would be an asymmetric smile which could last several weeks.

The Botox eyebrow lift

In the femininized face the brows arch above the brow bone whereas in a typical male face they sit lower. By selectively "freezing" some of the forehead muscles other muscles will pull harder than usual and, in this way, an arched brow can be formed.

The pout

By injecting very small amounts of Botox around the upper lip it can be possible to get a subtle relaxation of the muscles around the mouth. In some patients this can help "roll" the lips out. This technique is not for everyone, however. It takes a skilled injector as the muscles around the mouth are so important for eating, speaking and expression. Many patients also don't like the temporary weakness they can have which can affect their ability to suck through a straw and kiss.

Much more important for feminizing the lips are injectable fillers discussed later.

The Neck

Commonly used for anti-aging, the neck contour can sometimes improve with Botox. The platysma is a broad flimsy muscle that attaches to neck skin and can cause "banding" sometimes this is the reason behind a neck that is beginning to look saggy. By placing tiny amounts of Botox into the platysma muscle this can often help smooth out the neck.

Fillers

Fillers are substances that can be injected into the face to fill in different areas. They, like Botox can have great antiaging AND feminizing effects.

When we talk about fillers, a lot of people will mention collagen. In fact, collagen is very rarely used any more as a lot of patients developed allergies and it tended not to stay around for long.

Instead now there are a range of different brands and products that can be used to achieve different effects. One of the most common modern fillers is hyaluronic acid. In my practice, the majority of the results we are going to talk about can be achieved with this filler. Care must be taken when choosing an injector and a doctor is often best. Fillers are not without risks and the injector must be very familiar with the anatomy. Also, bad injections can cause bad deformities.

Anti-aging

Firstly, many patients seeking to feminize the face especially those over the age of 35 may benefit from the anti-aging effects of fillers.

Putting back volume

One of the earliest signs of aging is when the face begins to lose volume. This typically starts in most faces in the cheek area right under the pupil. Restoring this fullness can make the patient look less "tired" and youthful. It also can help smooth out the appearance of bags under the eyes.

Similarly, a sign of aging is sunken temples. By injecting fillers in this area a patient will look more youthful.

Brow enhancement

Brows are often overlooked but most faces lose fat earlier around the upper part of the eye socket.

Right above the pupil. When enough fat is lost, we can get a sunken appearance to the eye or an "a-frame deformity"

Carefully placed fillers can smooth this out and help give a more youthful feminized look.

Filling in lines

Deeper lines can also be improved with fillers. The "bracket lines" around the mouth also known as naso-labial folds can be smoothed and well as the "marionette lines" that extend down from the corner of the mouth and can give the patient the appearance that they are frowning all the time. The eleven lines or bunny lines that can't be softened with Botox should never, however be treated with fillers. In this area the risks are too high that the filler can make its way into the blood supply of the eye and even cause blindness. Fillers are best used for deeper lines and "folds". Fine lines are often better dealt with by using "resurfacing" techniques such as lasers and peels discussed later.

Certain fillers such as Sculptraâ are designed to help the overall quality of the skin – these can be injected widely in the face and neck and stimulate the body's own tissues to grow and fill in.

Improving cheek bones

An attractive feature, typically of a feminized face is strong high cheek bones. In fact, when we look at female faces from an oblique view an "ogee" curve or a "lazy s" shape is considered attractive.

We don't want to build up the whole face and create a "moon shape" but rather have a gentle curve or concave area underneath.

Fillers can certainly help build up the lateral cheeks to help create this appearance.

Liquid nose job

This has become a more common technique recently. However, all fillers can do is add to the nose. Overall usually to feminize the nose we want to make it smaller and more delicate. Sometimes some carefully placed filler at the tip of the nose can give the appearance of a more upturned nose which is a feature of a "feminine" nose.

Lips

So much can be achieved with fillers in the lips when it comes to feminizing the face. However, care must be taken to keep everything looking natural. It is possible to very significantly increase the size of the lips but the secret here is slow and steady. For many patients this usually means starting with at most one syringe to begin with. The lips can only increase in size a certain amount at a time or else we run into problems that come with distorting the anatomy such as lumpiness and an unnatural appearance.

Typically, most faces do best with the upper lip being 70% the size of the lower lip. The injector must also put the filler in the correct spot to make sure we don't create duck lips or visible lumps. It is important to find an experienced injector that can show you "before and afters". I emphasize this as lips are usually the most common thing I have to correct when it comes to fillers. It is possible to dissolve filler, but I have seen cases of really badly distorted lips that may never return fully to normal.

Typically, I recommend placing the filler just inside the lips into the area known as the dry wet border. This serves to plump out the vermillion or red part of the lip and doesn't interfere with the cupids bow. Most younger patients don't need any enhancement of the cupids bow and I believe it's usually best left alone.

The exception to this is more mature patients, especially smokers who have many vertical lines around the mouth. Filler at the cupid's bow can be important to smooth these out lines and rebuild the edge of the lip.

Lasers, Peels and Mechanical Resurfacing (Dermabrasion)

Improving the complexion and therefore softening the appearance of the skin can help in feminizing the face. There are a range of different ways that, to varying degrees can "resurface" the face and help reduce fine lines, scars and pigment giving a more even complexion. They can, to a lesser extent improve sagging skin. (however, surgery is usually required if this is significant). A discussion with your plastic surgeon will point you in the right direction of a procedure for your specific needs. Most techniques will require a series of treatments.

For the most effective and dramatic results these treatments may require anesthesia and significant "downtime" as the face becomes raw and heals from the treatment. With the more invasive treatments it may take the skin up to 4 weeks to return to normal.

These treatments may also be used at the same time as other surgeries depending on the needs of the patient.

Lasers – these can range from no down-time treatments (Including Intense Pulse Light) to ablative lasers such as Co2 lasers which remove the outer layers of skin and therefore can smooth lines and wrinkles.

Peels – Again depending on the type of acid used the outer damaged skin layer is removed to varying depths.

Mechanical Abrasion – In order to achieve similar goals, surgical scraping methods are used.

Hair removal

With time (up to 2 years) a combination of estrogen hormones and testosterone blockers will decrease hair density and coarseness. Many patients however may not find hormones alone adequate and therefore, many transfeminine patients will seek treatments for facial hair. Some studies have shown in fact, that this is the most common procedure transfeminine patients will undergo. Many patients may additionally be required to undergo hair removal for their planned gender affirmation surgery depending on the technique used.

Depilation just means plucking the hair – it can remove the hair for about 6 weeks and with repeated depilation over time it may result in damage to the hair bulb and decreased growth.

There are two main ways of "permanent" removal. No way is 100% effective though so they should be viewed at permanent hair reduction not removal.

Electrolysis is a method by which a needle is inserted to deliver current into the hair follicle and destroy it. It has to be done over hours and is quite painful often requiring numbing of some kind. It is recommended to be done on a weekly basis and can take many hours so can be very painful time consuming and expensive.

Laser hair removal has become more popular and is perhaps more effective. It is much less painful, and the typical length of treatment is 6 sessions at least 6 weeks apart. For many this is however the minimum. Many different types of light can be used by the laser to destroy hair follicles and whereas before it was only suitable for dark hair on light skin, more options are now available.

Skin Care for the transgender Woman

First know your skin

Hormones can have a tremendous effect on skin. In general, it is known that through a variety of mechanisms, estrogen has anti-aging effects on skin. Most plastic surgeons will include antiaging approaches when they perform feminizing procedures. A more "feminine complexion" typically means a smoother, wrinkle free complexion. So, what can we do to help achieve and maintain this at home? In this section we will discuss taking care of the trans-feminine complexion.

With transition, skin types can change

Skin types can be broadly classified into dry, oily or combination skin. With a decrease in sebum production as a result of decreased testosterone levels, a transitioning woman may notice her skin becoming drier gradually as the hormone levels change. Hormone replacement levels may also affect this. For example, dry skin on the other hand may be a sign that estrogens levels are on the lower side.

At home skin care routine

In order to better take care of skin it is important to have a good skin care routine in place.

I am a minimalist and I know the more steps a patient has to take the less likely she is to follow through.

In the cosmetics industry bold claims can easily be made without a shred of evidence to support them. I suggest rather than wasting money and effort on unproven treatments my patients just focus on what we know actually works.

This is my suggested routine

Morning

1. Cleanse (cheap cleansers are usually just fine. Foamy ones work well for oily skin)

2. Moisturize

3. SPF Sunscreen is critical year-round. At least SPF 30 is so important to decrease the aging effects of sunlight- don't forget to apply it to the back of the hands also!

Nighttime

1. Cleansing is more important at night to remove makeup and grime from the day

2. Moisturize

3. Antioxidant – My favorite on the market is Vitamin c products

4. Anti-aging – My favorite is Retinol

Exfoliation

This should happen every 3 days for oily skin and once a week for dry skin. Young skin turns over every 6 weeks whereas when we age this takes longer. Exfoliation can encourage this turn over and lead to a brighter complexion. This can be done with a facial scrub brush or a scrub product. Again, this is not something that has to be expensive in my opinion.

Vitamin C Products

These are my favorite types of antioxidants. Tissues can be susceptible to "oxidation" from a number of things in our environment and diets. Vitamin C is proven to help counter these aging effects. Not all vitamin C products are however created equally. Vitamin C quickly oxidizes when exposed to light so the container must be light proof. A lot of drug store products do not have a high enough concentration to be effective. This is therefore something worth investing in. Try to find products that have a concentration of 30%. Once the product turns brown it no longer works as it has oxidized.

Tretinion

This is a type of vitamin A that has a lot of evidence supporting its use. It has benefits when it comes to lines, wrinkles, pigment and even some evidence that it can decrease the chances of getting certain types of skin cancer. There are many retinol over the counter products available but most of the studies are done on tretinoin which is prescription only.

Most commonly patients can start out at 0.025% and advance to 0.05%. Many skin types are very sensitive initially to this product and it often causes excessive dryness and redness. Some patients must introduce it gradually perhaps even just 3 times a week at first. Over the course of the first one to two months the frequency can be increased to nightly.

Tretinion makes the skin very sensitive to sunlight so now more than ever sunscreen must be worn religiously.

Sunscreen

Tanning is one of the worst things we can do to age the skin. As mentioned before there is such overlap between anti-aging and feminizing treatments as a softer, youthful look signals feminine to the brain. Sunscreen needs to be worn daily and preferably year-round. At least factor 30 SPF with UVA and UVB protection. UVA rays age the skin while UVB rays burn the skin and both accelerate aging as well as the risk for skin cancers.

Lifestyle factors

In addition to above avoiding smoking, drinking enough water, eating a healthy balanced diet and excising will all help maintain a youthful complexion.

3. Bottom Surgery

By Sidhbh Gallagher

The first thing to understand about bottom surgery is – it is certainly not for everybody. Not all transgender women will want or need genital surgery in order to get relief from their gender dysphoria or to feel "whole". Therefore, it is important to know that there are different variations on vaginoplasty available.

Timing

The World Professional Association of Transgender Health produce standards of care which require that a patient be on at least 12 months continuously of hormone treatment and a year of full time living in their identity.

By the time patients reach their surgeon's office they have been waiting much longer. Understandably patients often have a sense of urgency about their surgery and factors such as waiting for insurance approval or surgery waiting lists can be incredibly frustrating.

This is however really a situation that the patient MUST be completely honest with herself and ask is now the right time?

Many patients admit that they underestimated the commitment a new vagina requires and how disruptive this procedure can be on both a physical and emotional level.

If a patient is not at a time in her life where she can meet the demands of post-op care real damage can be done. Without adequate emotional preparation breakdowns can happen and relationships can suffer. Without social and financial preparation jobs can be lost and funds run low. If the patient is unable to dilate after surgery for whatever reason vaginal depth will be lost perhaps permanently. Much of the recovery from vaginoplasty involves dilation. Regaining that depth is unreliable and risky business.

Your medical doctor and surgeon will help you decide if your physical health is where it needs to be (more about that later).

Many patients may elect to undergo a less demanding procedure to alleviate their dysphoria until they are at a point in life when they can undergo full vaginoplasty. Commonly patients will for example have an orchiectomy so that they can enjoy the hormonal benefits of this procedure until they are ready for full vaginoplasty. Happily, contrary to myths circulating the orchiectomy does not negatively impact future vaginoplasty.

How vaginas are created

Penile Inversion Vaginoplasty

This is the most common technique that is used in the United States to create a new vagina. In this operation the important parts of the penis -the pleasure nerves and most of the urethra (where the urine comes out) are saved along with the skin of the penis. The surgeon removes most of the tissue that gives erections (corpora cavernosa) and creates a new space to form a vaginal canal.

This canal is formed right underneath the **urethra** where the patient urinates from and right above the **rectum** where the bowel movements come from. This canal travels through the pelvic floor muscles.

Steps:

- The testicles and scrotal skin are removed, and the skin of the penis is turned inside out to create a new vagina and labia minora. Usually that extra scrotal skin will be used as a graft to create the deepest part of the vagina.

- The neo-clitoris (meaning new clitoris) is made from the head of the penis, which is greatly reduced in size but is designed to provide pleasurable sensation.

Fact: in some cases, these nerves may temporarily "go to sleep" after surgery but the vast majority of patients will regain great sensation.

The surgeon carefully preserves the nerves running to the head of the penis which are branches of the pudendal nerve.

Fact: Pudental nerve means the shame nerve in latin.

- The clitoris is placed above the urethra and a packing is placed inside the new vagina to stent it open during healing. The skin is then closed to form inner and outer vaginal lips. A tube (catheter) is kept in the bladder for about a week so the new urethra can heal.

This usually takes the surgeon somewhere between 3 and 5 hours.

<u>Fact: Depending on the surgeon, a rough estimate of the duration of surgery is "an hour per flaccid inch".</u>

The procedure described above is the most common way penile inversion is done. There are some variations -a common one is using parts other than skin to line the new vagina- either extra urethra or peritoneum. The idea behind these techniques is to try to make a vagina that lubricates itself. There isn't unfortunately evidence however, as yet, that either of these modifications make a difference.

Another modification, more commonly seen in Thailand and Europe is using the foreskin to create the inner labia. The foreskin is of course rarely available in the US for this technique.

<u>The "peritoneum" is a tissue that lines the inside of the abdominal cavity</u>.

Intestinal Vaginoplasty

Currently in the United States creating a vagina from the intestines is considered a secondary or back up procedure for patients who may have lost a previously created vagina.

Intestinal vaginoplasty involves taking a piece of bowel – usually colon and positioning it down into the pelvis to form a new vagina.

There are a few reasons many surgeons have moved away from using this method.

The appearance of the vagina made from intestine usually looks unnatural where it meets the skin. Intestine has a bright red color which, often does not blend well with the surrounding pink genitalia- patients call this the "stop sign" look.

It is unfortunately a myth that you don't have to dilate after this procedure. Its true that the intestine itself may not narrow as easily as a vagina made from penile inversion BUT there is often narrowing or "stenosis" where the intestine meets the skin.

Discharge can be a problem from the new vagina created from colon. One of the reasons patients may seek this procedure is that the new vagina "auto-lubricates". It can however be unpredictable how much it will produce, and patients may have problems with too much lubrication or even foul-smelling lubrication.

Longer recovery and morbidity. This procedure involves working inside the patient's abdomen, which can lengthen the patient's recovery and ability to start eating again after surgery. Usually the patient will require a longer hospital stay.

For these reasons this procedure is usually reserved as a "backup" procedure.

Peritoneal Pull Through Vaginoplasty

This procedure is a new approach in the gender affirmation surgery world but has been used in the gynecology world for years. About 1/5000 non-transgender women are born with "vaginal agenesis" meaning the vagina never forms and the peritoneum has been used to line the new vagina in these patients.

What, however, is the peritoneum? Inside the abdomen there is a membranous layer of tissue which lines the abdominal cavity. It is flimsy but a few different ways have been described to use it to line the new vagina.

Some surgeons have taken a piece out and used it as a graft- as in there is no blood supply and it must "take" like a graft. Others have used it to "cap" the penile inversion technique while still using penile and scrotal skin to line the lower parts of the vagina. In my practice we have tried to line as much of the new vagina as possible with the peritoneum that we get to with a robot.

The hope would be that unlike the penile inversion technique, where skin lines the new vagina, this membrane would line it instead and perhaps act more like a "natural" vagina.

Would this mean less dilation and more lubrication?

As yet we just don't know.

The downside to this technique is the patient needs cuts on the belly where the surgeon goes in to harvest the peritoneum. This opens up other potential risks as there are organs now close by to where we are working that could be damaged such as the intestines and ureters.

In my practice we have been able to almost completely line the new vagina with peritoneum. The first inch or so is still lined by the penile inversion skin. Therefore, there is no change in the outside appearance of the vagina.

Depending on how much of the peritoneum can be harvested (this depends on the patient's anatomy) more depth may be achieved.

Although there is a lot of interest in this technique only time will tell if the extra surgery is really worth it.

However, for patients who have been on blockers from an early age and do not have enough tissue to line a vagina this procedure may indeed be a better option.

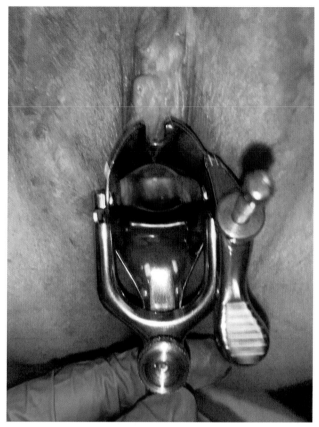

Figure 8 Patient with speculum in place showing the appearance of the peritoneal vaginoplasty.

One stage or two?

There is some debate over where vaginoplasty can be done all at once or in two separate procedures or stages. Most surgeons in the USA will try to do as much as possible at the first surgery –with the understanding that a percentage of patients may desire a labiaplasty at a later date.

Other Bottom Surgery Procedures

Orchiectomy

Some patients will choose to undergo just an orchiectomy by itself. This may be all the patient requires for their transition or they may not be at a point in their lives that they can deal with recovering from full vaginoplasty surgery.

<u>Fact; An orchiectomy will not interfere with later vaginoplasty</u>.

When the testicles are being removed for gender affirmation this is done through a small incision in the line that travels down the middle of the scrotum the "median raphè". An approximately 2-inch incision is all that's needed.

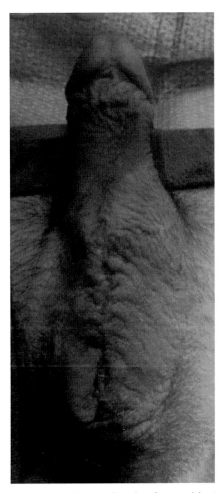

Figure 10 Patient immediately after orchiectomy.

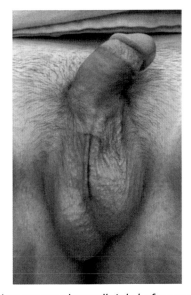

Figure 9 Appearance immediately before orchiectomy.

Scrotoplasty

This surgery is strictly for patients with no plans to have a vagina made in the future. It just means removal of the extra skin of the scrotum at the same time as removing the testicles. If a vagina is wanted some day, we need to save all the "spare parts" we can get. The scar is usually about 4 inches down the middle and doesn't add much to the recovery time from simple orchiectomy.

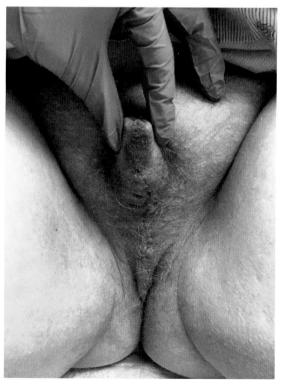

Figure 11 A patient one week after scrotoplasty which just requires a longer incision.

Figure 12 View of scrotoplasty incision.

Zero-depth or Dimple Vaginoplasty

This is a procedure where the genitalia are feminized in a very similar way to regular vaginoplasty. Just as in full vaginoplasty the testicles are removed as well as much of the scrotal skin and the penile erectile tissue. The urethra is shortened, and the head of the penis is formed into a neo-clitoris. However, instead of forming a skin-lined vaginal canal a dimple is just formed instead where the vagina would be.

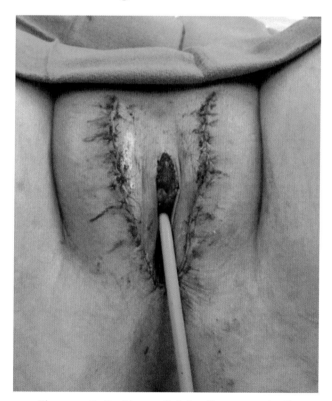

Figure 13 Patient immediately after a zero depth procedure.

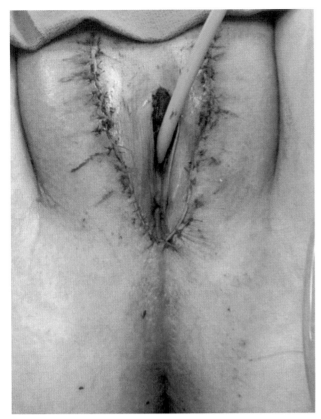

Figure 14 Instead of a vaginal canal a patient can choose to have a "dimple" of varying lenghts.

Patients chose this procedure for a few different reasons.

Most patients choosing this procedure identify as transfeminine.

In my practice often patients choosing this are attracted to women and have no interest in ever having penetrative intercourse.

This is a good option also for patients with a lot of medical co-morbidities as it shortens the recovery time and decreases the risks of various complications. Patients do not have to dilate afterwards.

In some patients creating a new vagina may have higher risks. An example of this would be a patient who has undergone previous prostatectomy (removal of the prostate usually for cancer). The area where the new vagina would be made is scarred so there is a higher risk of injuring the bowel or bladder.

Labiaplasty

A labiaplasty is an umbrella term which means any "nip-tuck" a patient may desire or need after their first bottom surgery to improve the appearance. The most common thing requested is a surgery to make the outer lips meet in the middle above the clitoris. (This is impossible at the first surgery as the blood supply to the vagina travels through here.) Other modifications can be done at this time to help improve the appearance – such as evening up the labia or maybe revising a scar.

Most surgeons will want to wait at least a few months after the first surgery before doing this part as the body will continue to improve upon the appearance as it heals, and the swelling reduces.

Before Labiaplasty

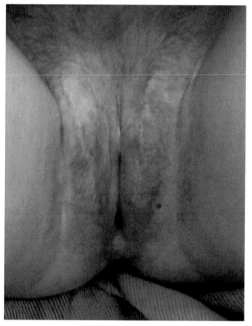

Figure 15 The LabiaMajora are separate in the pubic area.

After Labiaplasty

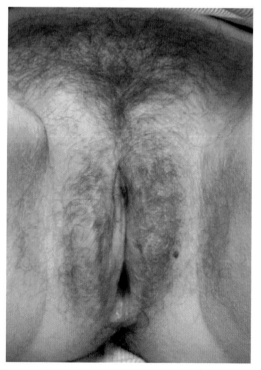

Figure 16 The Labia Majora are brought together at labiaplasty.

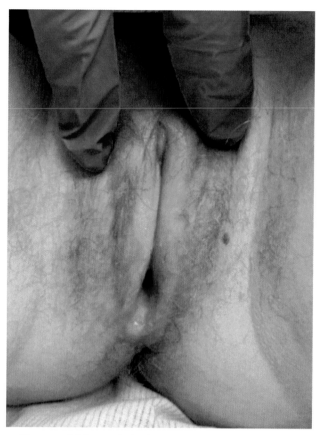

Figure 17 This can help form a more natural hooding over the clitoris.

What will my new anatomy look like?

There are huge variations in how a patient will look when she is finally healed from vaginoplasty just as there are huge variations in the appearance of any genitalia!

While I encourage a patient to bring pictures of how she would like to look, (preferably of transgender women) there is a potential for disappointment. Unfortunately, this situation is not like choosing from a menu -we can't simply select our favorite genitalia and make them appear! While the technique and surgeon style are certainly factors- probably the most important factor is the patient's own anatomy to begin with more specifically the quantity of skin or lack thereof.

A patient's preference is extremely important to me and in some respects (such as clitoral size) the patient can certainly have a say. Most patients will request that I "make things appear as natural as possible".

Certainly, as this surgery becomes more common in the United States many surgeons are committed to providing not only a safe functional result but also an aesthetically pleasing one.

Some modifications of the most commonly used penile inversion technique include using the foreskin to line the labia minora (commonly known in Thailand as the Chonburi flap). Of course, in the USA the foreskin is not usually available as most penises have been circumcised. In patients with smaller penises and not much scrotal skin (in the case of patients who have undergone treatment with blockers) skin grafts

may be required from the thighs, abdomen or groin.

Most surgeons will open up the patient's urethra in order to create the inner labia and provide a moist, pink area beneath or around the clitoris.

The degree of hooding of the clitoris after the first surgery depends on the availability of skin.

While we strive to create a symmetric appearance at the first surgery, asymmetries for example, caused by wound healing problems on one side can usually be corrected at labiaplasty

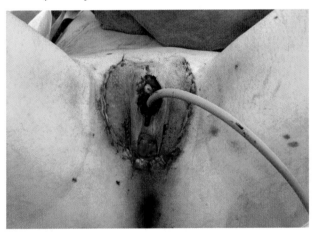

Figure 18 Patient immediately after undergoing penile inversion vaginoplasty. The appearance of the genitals will change a lot with time, and the patient may not see the final result for months.

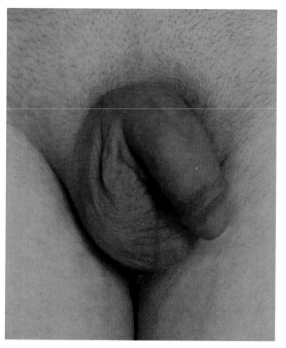

Figure 19 Patient before vaginoplasty.

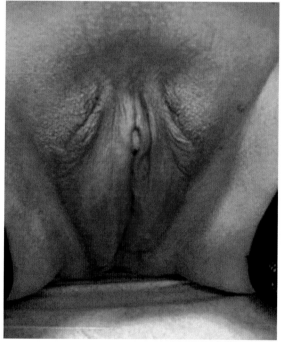

Figure 20 The same patient six weeks after vaginoplasty - the appearance of the genitals after surgery largely depends on the appearance before surgery.

Vaginoplasty- What can go Wrong?

Every surgery unfortunately carries a risk of things going wrong or complications.

When looking back at all the data from different studies Dr. Rumer and her research group found that approximately 32% of all patients will experience complications after this surgery. This number is likely higher as many studies may not include some of the annoying bumps in the road we will describe below.

With vaginoplasty patients will often experience "bumps in the road" as they heal (minor complications) while others will have more serious problems (major complications) which can indeed cause the patient to get ill, need another unplanned surgery or even have long-term problems. Nowadays surgery and anesthesia are remarkably safe (a long way from "the Danish Girl") so deaths from these procedures are extremely rare.

The Bumps in the Road (minor problems)

1. Wound Dehiscence

The most common complication a vaginoplasty patient may experience is wound dehiscence or wound separation. This is similar to "skin necrosis "' which means dead skin. In plastic surgery whenever we make a major rearrangement or change to a person's anatomy this has a higher likelihood of occurring. Depending on which study you read up to a third or more of patients will experience this. The good news is no matter how scary the wound may look when it opens up initially usually the powers of healing in the genital area are very impressive and these, sometimes ugly wounds, can heal almost without a trace over the next 2-3 weeks.

These wounds may look terrifying however there is usually not much extra pain caused by them. When we have a wound most of us want to slap a band aid on it and carry on with our lives while the body heals it. Unfortunately, the transgender vaginoplasty patient does not have this luxury!

Just around the time this scary looking wound is appearing in an already swollen distorted looking new vaginal area, a transgender woman should be dilating frequently. Often times this wound may be sitting right by the entrance to the new vagina or "introits" making the experience extra un-nerving!

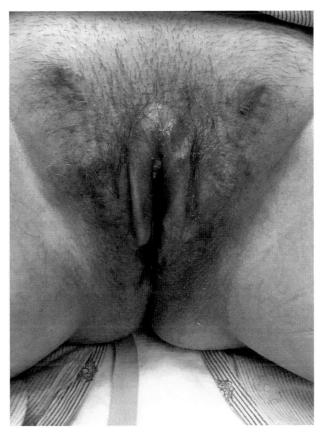

Figure 21 Patient with wound dehiscence and partial loss of the right labia minora. Small amount of yellowish tissue known as "exudate" on the clitoris.

How to fix the problem

The best antidote to this problem is time!

This is one of those "trust the process" moments. Your body will usually do a fantastic job of "healing-in" this open area without any long-term problems. Even if the area of skin loss is large usually the smartest approach is to allow the area to heal and much later any uneven-ness or unsightly scars can be taken care of at the time of labiaplasty (if a patient chooses to do this). I am still usually pleasantly surprised by how well things heal requiring no extra surgery at all.

Many patients are perplexed by why their surgeon won't just stitch up the area that has separated. As Einstein would say this would usually be an exercise in insanity- doing the same thing and expecting different results. Your body has shown us that it needs to heal in this way and therefore an interfering surgeon at this point will not help! Your body knows what it is doing- trust the process.

There ARE things a patient can do to help the process along, however.

Wound Care

Depending on the wound your surgeon may recommend some wound care. The approach we prefer is some antibiotic ointment. This helps prevent the area from becoming infected (it rarely does) and we know that open raw wounds like to be kept with a moist environment. If there is a lot of dead skin or "debris" or the typical yellowish exudate the surgeon may choose to gently remove this in the office to keep the area clean and encourage healing. Alternatively, the patient may help do this at home with

"sitz" baths or dressing changes. This should of course be done under the supervision of your surgeon or doctor.

Otherwise keeping the body happy and healthy is crucial at this time. Eat! A healthy balanced diet is critical to give the body the building blocks it needs to fill in these wounds. Unfortunately for many these wounds will be manifesting in the first 2-3 weeks after surgery when the patient is at risk of post-op depression.

If you are not eating, make sure your surgeon knows! It may be time to prescribe some supplements, as your wounds simply WILL NOT heal without these building blocks. Protein and a sensible diet are your friends at this point. If you are diabetic unfortunately your chances of wound healing problems are higher. During the recovery time keeping a good handle on those blood sugars will make a huge difference. Surgery or infection can make blood sugar more difficult to keep in check than usual so be sure to get help from a doctor if you are having difficulty controlling blood sugar.

Remember in general your doctor will advise you to KEEP DILATING during this time. As your body heals on the outside this is critical to maintain depth.

What NOT to do

Stay away from the substances that won't let your body do its job. Smoking at this time will have disastrous consequences for your healing. Nicotine will also be harmful. Even being around smokers and passive smoking is a huge "no-no". The same thing applies to smoking marijuana and most other drugs. Despite a patient's best intentions, the stress of surgery, recovery and post-op depression may cause a patient to relapse into bad habits. If you find yourself in this situation, it's time to get help. Irreversible damage can happen otherwise during this critical time of healing.

Vaginal Drainage

The new vagina is lined with (usually) a combination of skin from the penile shaft and the scrotum. On the inside a whole healing process is also taking place!

A patient will see evidence of this process in the form of vaginal discharge.

I tell patients that they can expect to wear maxi pads for the first 4-6

weeks after surgery. At first when the packing is removed, and the patient starts dilating she can expect to see bright red blood. Usually this spotting carries on for the first few weeks and it is indeed rare that she will get through a dilation session without at least seeing some blood tinged lube on her dilator. There are raw healing spots on the inside, which are causing this and are nothing at all to worry about.

Sometimes there may be some of that same skin necrosis or dead skin occurring on the inside of the new vagina. This time it will "slough" or peel off in its own time (often with the help of dilation or douching). It can give a yellowish stringy appearance to the drainage, which usually comes next.

If a patient develops a foul odor to the drainage or it gets copious this does however need to be checked out. Most commonly this problem can be taken care of by douching or sometimes an antibiotic gel or pills. Interesting fact is new vaginas rarely get yeast infections, as the PH is not conducive to it.

DO talk to your surgeon however as they will want to know about significant changes in the drainage to make sure that there is nothing more concerning at play.

Problems with Urination

Once the catheter (the tube that drains the bladder) comes out (this is usually 6-12 days after surgery) it is time to start urinating from your female anatomy!

If you are unable to urinate after the catheter is removed give your surgeon a call after a few hours this may be a sign that you have urinary retention. Up to 5% of patients may develop this when the catheter comes out at first. In general, its best if a patient does not go more than 8 hours without emptying their bladder. Do not fret if this happens to you. Usually a quick trip to the office or ER will take care of this. Most surgeons will choose to replace the catheter and probably try again in a week when there is less swelling.

Spraying is very common after vaginoplasty. Patients sitting to pee will often notice the stream hitting their thigh, the seat or even missing the bowl. Everything is still so swollen at this point and often once this swelling goes down this problem will resolve. This unfortunately can take months.

Patients may have "accidents" in the first few weeks and months after vaginoplasty – this usually means not making it to the bathroom in time. A patient may not make it to the bathroom on time (urge incontinence) or some leakage may happen when coughing or laughing stress incontinence). While about 16% of patients report this usually it settles down and most patients don't seek treatment. As the body adjusts after surgery this can be very frightening – but is rarely a permanent issue.

Urinary Tract Infections

The shorter the urethra the more likely the patient is to get a UTI.

Welcome to the world of having a shorter urethra! When you surgeon does your surgery, they usually shorten the urethra by about 4-5 inches. Urinary tract infections are more common in the first few weeks after surgery.

If a patient is having uncomfortable symptoms such as burning or stinging when she urinates, lower belly pain or having to go a lot may be signs of an infection. Tips to avoid it include always wiping from front to back and urinating after sex and dilation. Most primary care doctors will be comfortable treating a UTI in a transgender woman. However, it is very important for you to always remember that you do still have a prostate (a small one) but it also needs to be treated so this usually means some extra days (at least 10-14 days) on antibiotics. Therefore, your doctor NEEDS to know your anatomy in order to treat you correctly.

Strange feelings, numbness, pains

Pain after vaginoplasty overall is surprisingly not too bad for most patients. However, how much pain a patient feels after any procedure is a very personal thing. We now know that some patients simply don't respond as well to pain medications due to their genetics. In our practice, after typically 3 days in hospital patients will go home with prescription pain medications, which they are usually taking a few times a day. Once the packing comes out the patient will feel much more comfortable and typically, they will decrease their opiate medication down to just at night at about 2 weeks.

Feelings of numbness particularly around the incisions on the labia are very common and usually temporary as swelling decreases and the skin heals so will normal sensation return. In addition, it is common to have some numbness of the clitoris usually just limited to one side. This too almost always gets better.

As the nerves in the area "Waken up" patients may report a dragging sensation or sometimes little jolts and shocks of sensation. For most these are gone at 3 months. For others we have found that pelvic floor physical therapy can be highly effective at relieving these symptoms.

Bruising, swelling and granulation tissue

The appearance of the area will change drastically in the first few months. In fact, from what a patient looks like in the days following surgery to her appearance at 6 months to a year is almost unrecognizable.

Because as humans we spend most of our time in an upright position "down there" is usually the most "dependent" or lowest part so it swells. It swells A LOT usually for weeks and months after the surgery.

Initially when you start to explore your new anatomy the clitoris often will be obscured by a very swollen mons and the labia minora have little definition they are so swollen. It is not until 6 weeks or more that things slowly start taking shape.

Some patients will have more bruising than others and often it can be asymmetrical causing further worries about the future appearance.

My advice again here is to trust the process put the mirror down and be assured that how things look initially are nothing like they will look when the swelling goes away.

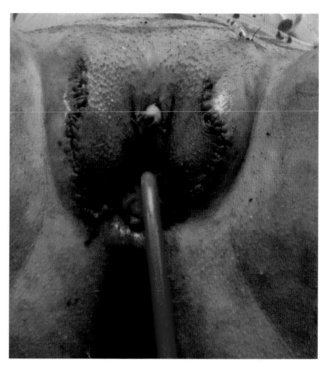

Figure 22 Swollen appearance right after surgery.

Granulation tissue is a process by which the body heals maybe a little too much – it forms raised fleshy areas that are usually bright red and easily bleed. This tissue is common around the urethra and the opening of the vagina. It actually can cause some discomfort in many patients. The treatment is usually to cauterize it in order to shrink it. Often your surgeon will do this easily and painlessly in the office.

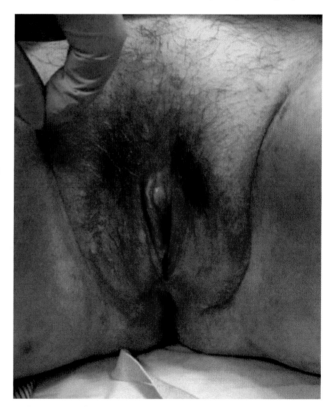

Figure 23 A few months later the appearance is almost unrecognizable.

Serious Complications

Complications can happen with vaginoplasty that can require another unplanned surgery or may even lead to permanent issues.

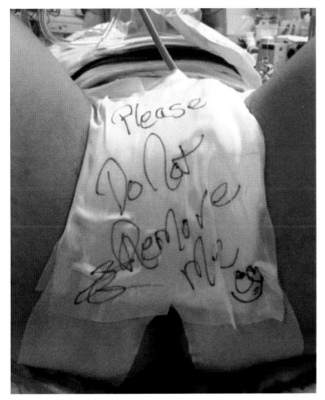

Figure 24 Patient right after vaginoplasty - in our practice a tight pressure dressing is left on for the first few days to help avoid bleeding.

Bleeding

In the early post-operative phase, the complication we worry about most is bleeding. Blood loss is inevitable with vaginoplasty and your surgeon will want to make sure you are not anemic by checking a standard hemoglobin (blood count) prior to surgery. Surgery may even be delayed if it's not where it should be to start out.

The most likely time for bleeding is in the first 24-48 hrs. In order to help prevent that your surgeon will place a compressive dressing after surgery either sewn or snuggly taped into position and take other measures such as keeping your blood pressure from creeping too high. The good news is this bleeding most commonly comes from the new urethra on the outside so it's rarely internal bleeding requiring more surgery. Usually your surgeon can handle this at the bedside without the need for an emergency surgery. Serious bleeding requiring a blood transfusion according to the literature happens less than 1% of the time.

Recto-neovaginal fistula

Most would agree the trickiest part of this surgery is creating a new vagina cavity, safely creating a canal where none was present before. The new vagina is created right between where the prostate is and the rectum.

A recto- neovaginal fistula is perhaps the most worrisome problem after vaginoplasty. What it means is an abnormal connection or "fistula" going between the rectum, which stores the stool and the new vagina (neovagina). The problem with this connection is the stool now leaks out of the new vagina instead of staying in the rectum where it belongs.

This is usually thought to happen either when the rectum is injured or weakened at the time of surgery or perhaps through dilation after surgery. This complication luckily only happens in 1-2% of patients. When it does happen however, one or more surgeries are required to fix it. It will also take time, time away from work and a patient's life, which is unexpected and often extremely upsetting. Fixing it may also require temporarily diverting the stool away from the area you are trying to heal. This means creating a temporary "stoma" or "ostomy" on the abdomen – so the patient must wear a bag during that time. The priority becomes healing the rectum so keeping the new vagina can be a real challenge. Many surgeons will have a patient stop dilating at this time so as not to make the abnormal connection or fistula worse and once everything is healed then focus on regaining vaginal depth. Unfortunately, after a problem like this a lot of scarring will be present and it may be necessary

if the new vagina has scarred over to recreate it with another method such as using intestine.

Urinary/meatal stenosis

When the anatomy is feminized the urethra is shortened and repositioned. It is possible that during the healing process some scaring may take place, which can narrow the urethra, usually at its opening. There can be scarring of the new labia over the area or scaring of the urethra itself. This can lead to difficulty urinating and may require another surgery with temporary re-insertion of the catheter to allow it to heal. This problem usually happens about a month after surgery and patients typically report frequent urination, difficulty getting a stream started and waking up at night to urinate. This complication is reported at up to 15%.

Vaginal Stenosis

This problem is reported at 5% but is likely much, much higher in my opinion. This is why we surgeons are constantly preaching the importance of dilation after vaginoplasty. It's an unfortunate fact that when it comes to neovaginas it's a case of "use it or lose it". This seems to be the case with ANY new vagina – many studies have shown that intestinal vaginas will also narrow at the entrance without dilation. Dilation will be needed forever (although sexual intercourse counts). Depth is more important to maintain than girth. This is why when dilating we always recommend when the dilator is all the way in putting some gentle pressure on that back wall to keep it open. Girth can be dialed up later more easily just by using dilators, but depth can be difficult to regain.

Every patient is different in how much they can "get away" without dilating and still maintain an open vagina. It is generally recommended that during the maintenance phase (once everything is healed) a schedule of about 3 times a week is recommended. Patients should however increase the frequency if she notices things getting tighter.

In some cases, if a patient has healing problems at the entrance of the vagina – even despite of her best efforts with dilation – narrowing of the opening of the vagina may happen which often requires a surgery to correct.

In my experience – patients who developed stenosis usually had abandoned dilation for weeks or months at a time. A surgery is often required to reopen the narrowed vagina and the patient usually has to return to the same intensive dilation schedule as after the very first surgery as that reopened vagina will be at more risk than ever of scarring back down. In some cases, scarring may be so severe that a reconstruction with another vaginoplasty method may be necessary.

Unfortunately, anytime we operate in a scarred field the anatomy is distorted and all the other risks of surgery, in particular the recto-neo-vaginal fistula, is much more likely to occur.

Therefore, dilation as prescribed by your surgeon is of critical importance in taking care of the new vagina.

Later Complications

As healing continues after vaginoplasty, most of the more serious complications listed above become less of a concern. However, some other bothersome problems may arise.

Problematic Swelling with Arousal

As the swelling from vaginoplasty subsides in the first few months some patients may notice swelling with arousal. This is to be expected as all genitalia male and female have "erectile" tissue. In the case of vaginoplasty there will be erectile tissue around the new clitoris as well as a variable amount around the urethra.

With modern techniques the majority of the corpora cavernosa (the main erectile bodies) will have been removed so they don't usually contribute much to swelling.

The corpora spongiosum however is the erectile tissue that is wrapped around the urethra itself. It varies a lot from patient to patient how much of this is present. In patients who have more, a patient may notice swelling usually on one side more than the other when she is aroused. Rarely the swelling may push down from above on the vagina and even block the entrance making penetration difficult.

Usually this problem can be solved by removing the extra tissue (usually at the time of labiaplasty). It can be helpful to have pictures of the offending swelling to show your surgeon and help guide her in the operating room when removing it.

This is usually a relatively easy outpatient procedure; however, a catheter may be needed as the patient recovers.

Labial Adhesions

Sometimes, especially if there were wound healing issues initially at the time of surgery, the labia minora may cause problems as they heal in. A common issue is labial adhesions or agglutination. It may be possible for the labia to fuse together as they heal. If your surgeon suspects this may be happening, they may prescribe topical estrogen creams. In the long run this may not cause any issues. It can lead to less well-defined labia minora or in more severe cases possibly block the opening of the urethra or fuse over the clitoris. Oftentimes this can be addressed at the time of labiaplasty. It is usually a relatively easy outpatient surgery. A catheter may be needed however during recovery.

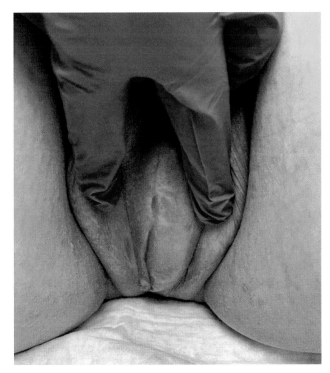

Figure 25 A patient a year after penile inversion vaginoplasty who developed labial adhesions.

Sensation Problems

After a major surgery and rearrangement of the anatomy it can take many months for the nerves to get back to normal. As a general rule most patients who could orgasm before surgery will eventually be able to orgasm again.

Sometimes there may be numbness around the clitoris. The dorsal nerves which previously supplied the head of the penis may take several months to fully function again. This is known as a neuropraxia where they temporarily "go to sleep". While it may take many months and a lot of patience for them

to wake up it is very rare to have permanent loss of the nerves on both sides. As mentioned elsewhere it can take some time to figure out what works well to stimulate the new anatomy.

On the other end of the spectrum sometimes too much sensation can be present. Patients may feel a sensation of always being aroused and certain types of underwear or positions may cause irritation. For the majority of patients this will be mild and transient. In addition, as the nerves "wake up again" many patients will describe "lightning- bolt" type sudden sensations in the genitalia that usually pass quickly. In rare cases if this discomfort, hypersensitivity or irritation continues, it may be necessary to seek treatments. Types of physical therapy can help with the unusual sensations and some drugs are available to "calm down" the over acting nerves. Time usually cures all patients who have these issues.

The countdown to Surgery

How best to prepare your body for your new vagina?

The biggest change vaginoplasty poses to a patient's body is that there is a lot of wound healing to do afterwards.

The healthier a patient is before vaginoplasty the smoother her recovery will likely be. It is best if a patient begins to prepare herself for this major surgery early on particularly if she is not in the best shape.

Nutrition

Vaginoplasty of course involves a major rearrangement of a patient's anatomy

Keeping a healthy weight is critical prior to surgery. Many surgeons will have BMI requirements prior to undergoing surgery. (Discussed elsewhere.) For most this will be a BMI of less than 30-35 and over 18. Your body needs the building blocks to heal after surgery, so this means crash dieting around the time of surgery is a no-no. If a patient has succeeded in losing a lot of weight prior to surgery she will want to be out of that weight loss phase and in the "maintenance phase" prior to surgery. This is especially important when a patient has undergone a weight loss surgery.

Some blood tests to check the building blocks are present are usually prudent. These blood tests include a hemoglobin to check for anemia and pre-albumin to check protein levels. Some patients may be found to have a low hemoglobin before surgery. Often times this will have to be investigated and treated before surgery.

Other Medical Conditions

Anemia

The most common reason we see behind the low hemoglobin or anemia is iron deficiency. Once this cause has been established and other causes ruled out the surgery may need to be postponed until the hemoglobin improves. While we try to limit blood loss as much as possible from this surgery starting out with low hemoglobin increases the chances of needing a blood transfusion afterwards.

Diabetes

Diabetic patients will require a test called the Hemoglobin A1c to check how well sugars are being controlled. Target levels are usually 7 or less in order to allow best wound healing.

Smoking

Smoking is about the most harmful practice around the time of vaginoplasty. We are performing a major rearrangement of the tissue and therefore some of that rearranged tissue will have much less of a blood supply until everything is healed. We know that every time a cigarette is smoked this blood supply is further cut off and a process called tissue necrosis or death is inevitable. What this means is that large areas of the new genitalia will literally "die off" (as scary as that sounds) and open wounds for prolonged periods and scarring are inevitable.

Unfortunately, any product that contains nicotine (sorry vapes, patches and even gum) can have this dangerous effect on wound healing. Smoking marijuana seems to be just as dangerous for wound healing as cigarettes.

How long do I need to stop?

The magic number we talk about in surgery is that a patient stops smoking for at least 6 weeks before a surgery and 6 weeks afterwards. I'm not a fan of this as most patients do manage to kick the habit for good once they are able to stop for 3 months! Picking up smoking again at 6 weeks may well cause a lot of damage anyway.

Stay away from other smokers. It has been shown that passive smoking or inhaling the smoke from other's cigarettes can be just as dangerous or even worse than the patient themselves smoking.

Smoking is a deal breaker for vaginoplasty- some surgeries may be reluctantly done on smokers – this is not one of them. Many surgeons will ask the patient to provide a urine sample to show the nicotine is out of their system prior to surgery and indeed cancel them if it's not.

Heart and Lung problems

If a patient has other serious health issues, they will require some more investigation before surgery. In collaboration with the anesthesiologists and possibly the patient's heart or lung specialist we work to "risk stratify" the patient. This means figuring out how safe it is to move forward with surgery. If the patient has had a recent issue such as a heart attack or pneumonia most providers will want to get the patient fully recovered in order to undergo surgery.

Being under anesthesia for 4-5 hours is tough on the body so it is critical that the patient is safe to proceed.

Bleeding Problems

There are many different conditions a patient may have that make them prone to bleeding. In this case the surgeon will usually work closely with the patient's hematologist (blood doctor) to ensure the patient is kept as safe as possible. Often times medications can be used around the time of surgery to help decrease the risks. This may mean longer in hospital and perhaps an increased chance of bruising swelling or blood transfusion.

Clotting disorder

There are many reasons a patient may be at higher risk than usual for developing blood clots after surgery. The concern is the patient can start by developing a "deep vein thrombosis" which ultimately could travel to the lung and even be fatal. Patients who have previously been diagnosed with a condition that increases their risk may often be on blood thinners full time. These will usually have to be stopped for a time around surgery and then restarted when felt safe to do so. The surgeon will usually want to liaise with the patient's hematologist in order to make a

plan to carry out the procedure and recovery period safely.

HIV

Being HIV positive is not a reason not to have surgery. HIV positive patients who have optimized CD4 counts will do just as well as any other patient. Up to date blood work will be checked and the surgeon may liaise with the patient's infectious disease team in order to ensure the patient is in the best possible shape for surgery.

Prostate issues

If a patient has undergone previous prostate surgery (in particular for prostate cancer) or radiation, the area where the new vagina is to be formed will be scarred. What this usually means is the patient has a much higher risk than normal of an injury to the rectum. Depending on the patient's situation it may be recommended that the patient undergo the safer option of a "zero depth" procedure. This way the risks of surgery are a lot less.

Hair Removal /Reduction

Performing a Penile Inversion vaginoplasty means using hair-bearing skin to line the new vagina. This in particular refers to the scrotal skin which will go on to become the deepest part. Right now, patients will opt for laser or electrolysis to do this.

Laser hair removal

This is a process which involves using a specialized laser to target the hair follicles and destroy them one by one. Traditionally it was best in the setting of dark hairs and light skin. As technology has advanced more fair-haired patients can opt for this. It is done with the patient awake, takes about 10 minutes a session and at a very minimum needs to be done six times, six weeks apart. The discomfort is like an elastic band being flicked against the skin every time. It is more widely available.

Electrolysis

This is less widely available but considered more thorough than laser. The patient will undergo "hours "rather than sessions. It is painful and some centers will offer either local or full anesthesia for this.

Why are Multiple Cycles Needed?

The hair cycle requires that many sessions of hair removal may be necessary as a hair must be present at the time of the session in order to destroy the follicle. Hairs have a cyclical lifecycle meaning they will intermittently not grow, and "sleep" known as the "telogen phase".

Controversy

This is one of the more controversial topics in gender affirmation surgery leading some surgeons to advise their patients it's an absolute must and other who don't insist on it and therefore some very confused patients.

Let's take a look at the arguments for both.

Pro Hair removal

1-If a patient has problems with hair growth in the vagina it's almost impossible to treat.

2- This is elective surgery in that the patient has time to use one of these modalities before surgery

Against Hair removal

1- it is painful, expensive, can be difficult to find a culturally competent laser or electrolysis practitioner. Having the genitals that are such a source of dysphoria exposed and worked upon for long periods of time can be even psychologically traumatic for some patients. This is one of the more significant barriers to bottom surgery I have seen in practice.

2-In my opinion hair removal is a misnomer, I have never seen complete clearing of follicles in even the most treated patients. It is hair reduction.

A patient survey of 232 patients who had undergone penile inversion vaginoplasty reported that only 7% of patients had significant problems with hair growth after surgery. Whether or not a patient had undergone hair removal prior to surgery made no difference in whether she had problems post-operatively.

What to do?

When making decisions about our practice a lot of things are decided by surgeons from "dogma" as in we do unquestioningly things because this is "how it's always been done" or how we were trained. Every surgeon knows the better approach is to do things based on evidence and documented experience. There unfortunately is a real lack of evidence to answer many questions in gender affirmation surgery. Based on what IS in the literature and speaking to other very busy surgeons, I have changed my recommendation to patients. While

hair reduction prior to surgery is always preferable, I have removed it as a barrier to surgery for my patients. During the surgery we meticulously remove follicles from the underside of the scrotal graft with cautery. There are limitations to this as mentioned earlier as some of those follicles may be "hiding" in telogen phase. So far, I have found this a safe approach for patients.

The Bowel Prep

When the plan is to create a new vagina, many surgeons will insist on a pre-operative "bowel prep". This is when laxatives and antibiotics are given to make the bowels as "clean" and "cleared out" as possible prior to surgery. The theory is if the worst happens and an injury to the bowel occurs having a "clean", "stool-free" as possible environment will help if your body needs to repair it.

From a practical standpoint the patient will need to be prepared for what the bowel prep involves.

For the day before surgery and into the night she will need quick access to a rest room. Therefore, travelling in the on day before surgery is a bad idea. If a patient is local, she should plan on taking the day before surgery off work also.

In my practice, based on literature from Japan we do not insist on a bowel prep any longer. In that study they looked at patients undergoing removal of the prostate (similar risk for injury to the rectum) and asked does bowel prep help when the rectum gets injured? When creating a new vagina, we work in the same area and therefore have the same risks. They found however that the bowel prep made no difference to the patient's outcomes when they did get a rectal injury.

Your Hospital Bag – what to pack!

What you will need will vary greatly from facility to facility. If you are funding your own surgery, it will likely be done in an outpatient setting and usually your doctor will give you a very specific list of must-haves such as a donut pillow to keep pressure off when you sit or stockings to help prevent blood clots.

If you are in the hospital settings often most things will be provided.

You do however need your preferred toiletries, and the essentials such as a phone charger. A good book or your journal may also be very helpful.

Keep in mind you will need a practical going home outfit. When released from the hospital there will usually be a catheter still attached. This is usually connected to a leg bag. Therefore, skinny jeans are out. Think loose floaty clothing like long skirts or loose sweatpants.

Secondly many surgeons will send you home with either a maxi pad or somewhat bulky dressing. Loose comfy "granny-panties" that you don't care about staining are the best choice during these early days.

A pack of these maxi pads will be very useful to have for the trip home. Staining and sometimes oozing are common.

Thinking ahead

Just for practical reasons alone – this is not a process a patient can go through by herself. There needs to be SOMEBODY available to help afterwards and this isn't even taking into consideration all the emotional support that will be needed. If right now nobody is available, that means surgery needs to be pushed back a little while until somebody is available.

In the weeks after surgery a patient driving herself is not possible. This is because she will be on strong painkillers, which make it illegal and she will be somewhat disabled and perhaps not able to make the necessary sudden movements after surgery that driving may require.

The earliest patients will return to driving is 2 weeks after surgery. Often times about 2 doctor visits will be needed during this time.

It's important to plan ahead to have healthy food available after surgery. In the days and weeks following the surgery a healthy diet is critical to give the body the many building bricks it needs to heal.

Also prior to surgery stock up on maxi pads/sanitary towels, water-based lube and one or more douche kits.

Planning your recovery

Vaginoplasty even when covered through insurance, is financially demanding.

Keep in mind everything going smoothly 6 weeks are required off work. After this, sitting for prolonged periods of time may be difficult and a patient will need to have access to privacy for probably at least one dilation during the working day.

It is important to speak with HR and be clear about what exactly the plan will be, what paperwork for example short term disability is needed and whether or not maybe a "work from home" or light duty option is available.

Think about trips back to see your surgeon and follow-up care. Can you afford them? If not will your primary care doc or maybe a gyn take over?

Think ahead also will there be another stage to this surgery? A labiaplasty? In the days of high deductible insurance plans. Trying to fit these 2 procedures into the same calendar year can save a patient a lot of money. Therefore, vaginoplasty may be advantageous in the first part of the year.

It is wisest to postpone other big life events such as weddings or vacations for about 3 months after surgery. By this time the majority patients will be recovered enough.

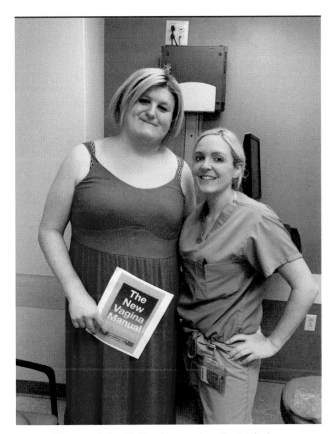

Figure 26 Dr. Gallagher and patient Kimber.

The New Vagina Manual

Introduction

The days and weeks after surgery can be pretty scary and confusing for patients. There is a whole new world of sensations and emotions to get used to. Some very unexpected feelings both physically and emotionally can sneak up on you. Your emotional recovery is JUST as important as the physical.

We got tired of telling our post-op vaginoplasty patients "it doesn't come with a manual" so here it is – The Manual -what to expect after bottom surgery. Please note that is is what we recommend for OUR patients. Every surgeon may vary a little (or a lot) in their technique and post-op instructions so it is critical to listen to your specific surgeon. These are provided for educational purposes only.

new vagina will change drastically over the first year. Indeed, it may be completely unrecognizable when the swelling goes down so Do Not fret if things look strange on first inspection.

Here is a what the new vagina *might* look like a few months into recovery. Again, I emphasize every patient will look different

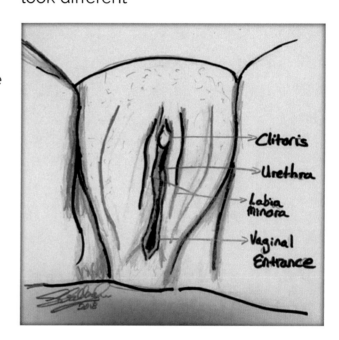

Your New Anatomy

The new you

The appearance of every patient's anatomy is unique to her, it is determined largely by what her anatomy was like before. It is critical to remember the appearance of the

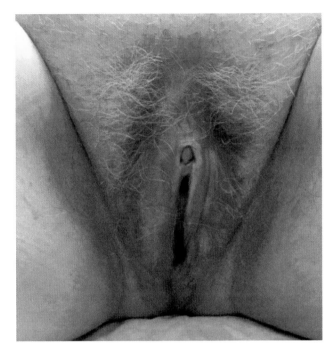

Clitoris; once was head of the penis. This may be pretty hidden until the swelling comes down. A little numbness usually on one side or the other is common until things heal. Like any clitoris there is more erectile tissue underneath the skin so swelling in this area is common when you are turned on. This is the center of pleasure for most women.

Urethra; previously longer, this is where you urinate from. It's the most common culprit if you get bleeding in the early days after surgery.

Labia Minora; once was penile skin. Every woman's labia look different, in the first few months after surgery they may not be clearly visible due to swelling but often appear as the swelling goes down.

Labia Majora; once was scrotal skin. Usually, the scars are hidden in about the middle of the labia majora. It is very common to have a lot of numbness here in the early weeks of healing.

Vaginal entrance: this is the most common place to get wound healing problems but usually the scars fade very well here. Sometimes the scars may cause narrowing of the entrance which your surgeon may have to address.

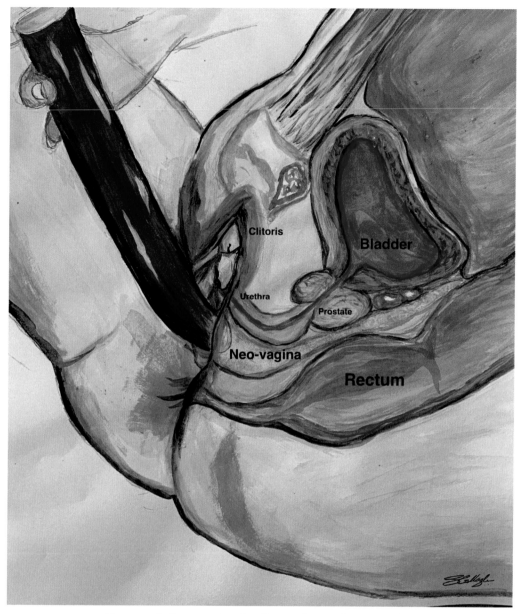

Figure 27 A diagram showing the anatomy of a neovagina.

Dilation

First rule of dilation is RELAX in every sense of the word. This process is entirely for you. It should not be scary or painful. This is your vagina! You are in charge!

Why dilation?

Your new vagina is created in a space that was not previously there and lined with your own tissue. Your body is very good at healing itself and will always try to close down this space if the new vagina isn't used- this means either using a dilator or having sex.

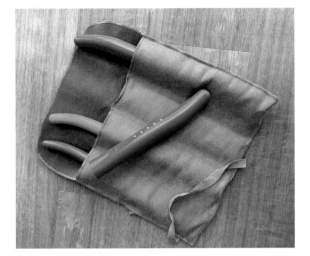

Figure 28 Typical set of dilators form Soul Source LLC.

How to dilate

Dilation much be taught by an expert. Do not attempt to use these instructions to learn by yourself. Follow YOUR surgeon's instructions. These are provided to educate as to what our patients do only.

Before you begin to use a dilator, it is very important to be as relaxed as you possibly can. Each person is different so it is beneficial to experiment with relaxation methods to find which is suitable for you, these may include soothing music, ambiance, warm bath, meditation or guided imagery. The more focused you are the more successful you will be. Remember the dilator is your friend; its only function is to help you.

Using your dilator:

1. **Positioning** - Lie on your back with your knees bent, propping pillows may help-your comfort is everything. Towels are helpful as lube can get messy and spotting of blood is typical in the first few weeks.

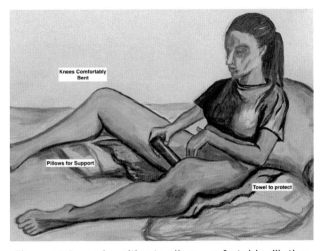

Figure 29 A good position to allow comfortable dilation.

2. **Lubricant** - This should be water-soluble and free of glycol. Cover the dilator in lubricant.

3. **Mirror and lighting**- the first few weeks of dilating require good lighting and a mirror until you get a feel for your new anatomy.

4. **Inserting the dilator**-Always start with the smallest dilator recommended by your surgeon. Often the vagina follows a curved shape, so you are going in and up with a forward direction. (see

diagram below – this is because of the shape of the bulbospongiosum -erectile tissue-left around the urethra). Tip is up and you are aiming for your belly button. Carefully slide the tip of the dilator in, take your time and focus on how you feel. As long as your discomfort is no greater than 3 out of 10 slowly continue to insert the dilator. Take frequent breaks holding the dilator in position, when you feel ready slide it in a little further. Sometimes a gentle side-to-side wriggling may help.

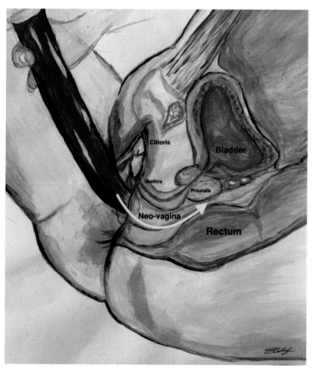

Figure 30 Diagram of the anatomy showing why a "scooping" motion of the dilator is usually needed when entering the neovagina.

4. Once it is in, hold the dilator in a position that does not increase discomfort above 3 or 4 out of 10. Putting small amount of pressure on the dilator during this time will help keep the deepest part of your vagina open. Keep your dilator in for 15 minutes or move up to that next size if ready and cleared to do so.

5. When moving to the next size repeat the process as above making sure all the while that the discomfort does not stay above a maximum of 4 out of 10. However, if the pain momentarily reaches 6 and quickly back drops to 2 out of 10, this is ok. Remember don't freak out if you can't do the larger dilator today – there will be good days and bad days and some days you will be more swollen than others.

6. What you are aiming to do is progress through dilator size at a pace which is comfortable for you (this can vary from weeks to months depending on the individual) so that you are able to use your goal dilator without discomfort greater than 3-4 out of 10. Remember this is YOUR goal dilator it DOES NOT have to be the largest dilator in the pouch.

Top Tips

a) Expert dilators know that dilation can and really should become fun "me time" when you take the time to learn what feels good and maybe even incorporate the occasional orgasm into your routine. As you progress, having a partner assist in using the dilators, or using them as part of foreplay or transition to sexual intercourse, can also make the experience more fun.

b) Experimentation with different leg or trunk positions can result in greater comfort, exploring different angles of insertion can also prove beneficial.

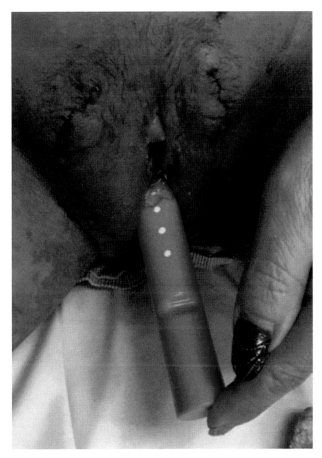

Figure 31 First dilation

c) Don't let that brightly colored stick of plastic ruin your day. If it's not going in relax and try later or even call it a day. Skipping a day or even 2 early in your recovery is ok. You are in charge here! This should NOT be painful or stressful. The good news is penetrative intercourse counts as dilation.

d) If you are dealing with a painful or swollen vagina most dilators can be popped into the freezer to cool them off. This can give some relief like an internal "cooling pad".

Sample Schedule

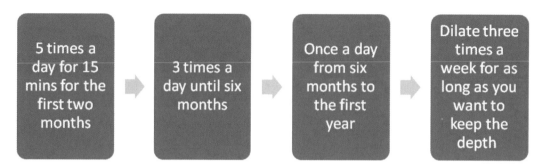

5 times a day for 15 mins for the first two months → 3 times a day until six months → Once a day from six months to the first year → Dilate three times a week for as long as you want to keep the depth

Remember; In the beginning, in particular, there will be good days and bad days. If you are having an off day with dilation it is a good strategy to go as deep as you can, following the steps above, with the skinniest dilator. You can always gain back width more easily than depth later.

How big do I need to go?

This is the BIG question – does size matter?

A lot of our patients struggle with feeling like they are "underachievers" in the early days of dilation because that monster dilator looks like it will never go in.

Remember you are the BOSS.

The average length of a cis-gender vagina is 9cm or 3.5inches (this may be longer when aroused according to some studies). Most studies show that the average length of a transgender vagina is about 10cm or 3.9inches. Women and their partners don't seem to have difficulty with sex unless the vagina is less than 7cm or 2.7 inches. Therefore, in gynecology a 7cm vagina is considered small but still normal.

So how big do you need to be? The answer totally depends on what you plan to use your vagina for. In most cases, if you are planning to have penetrative sex, it depends on how large your partners penis is. Match that to the dilator and there's your answer! There is no need to go bigger than this although many patients will do so to help relieve anxiety at first during sex.

Upsizing

Upsizing your vagina (within reason) is possible DO NOT underestimate the power of dilation. Studies have shown that with slow and steady persistence inches can be gained with dilation alone. Therefore, a larger partner may indeed be accommodated in time. Pelvic floor physical therapists can help design a schedule to get to your goal.

Sticking to the dilation schedule is critical so as to prevent scarring which may need a major surgery to reverse. If you do need a surgery to open things back up eventually it can be riskier than the first surgery as there is a lot of scar tissue and therefore injury to the bladder or bowel may be a bigger concern.

Sex

Orgasm

This is often the exciting and fun part of recovery from your vaginoplasty! Exploration and masturbation are encouraged whenever you feel well enough to do so. For most patients this is at about 2 weeks at the earliest. This is the time to learn what feels good and what you need to become aroused. When you are ready this can be incorporated into your usual dilation routine whenever time and mood permit!

Initially one of the first things patients will notice when they get aroused for the first-time during recovery is the swelling of the tissue. There is some erectile tissue present (just as there is in a cisgender vagina) and so when turned on the clitoris and some surrounding tissue will enlarge. DO NOT worry –you will not do any harm. It can be achy and unpleasant if this is early in recovery – if that is the case take a Tylenol and think of something else!

Sexual response varies so much among women and there are many factors involved other than just anatomy- emotions, relationships hormones as well as overall health and wellness.

For most post-op patients, the most sensitive area is the new clitoris. Like any clitoris direct touching and pressure may be too intense so experiment. For example, many patients may find directly touching that area with a vibrator too much. In early recovery the nerves there are re-adjusting and as such some patients may experience some numbness or oversensitivity in the first few weeks – this will get better.

In addition, the prostate which is still there can be stimulated through the new vagina perhaps similar to the "G spot" – many transgender women find this can also provide pleasure. This is located on the front wall of the vagina usually a couple of inches in. Dilation sessions can be a good time to find this area either with a finger or dilator and experiment with what feels good to you.

Oral sex/Foreplay/Fingering

At about 4 weeks as long as you are healed and feeling ready it is safe to start experimenting with what feels good with your partner on the outside. Most of your sexual pleasure will come from the new clitoris so it's a good time to start finding out what feels good and works for you. Remember however not all patients will be ready at 4 weeks.

Penetration

You won't be ready to entertain a penis until you are completely healed which is about 8 weeks or sometimes longer.

The same applies for anal sex. The new vagina lives right next door to the anus so waiting at least 8 weeks is safest to prevent injury.

Slow and steady is key here and you must be completely comfortable with dilators before taking on a live penis!

With any good sex it is key that you know what feels good to you so that you can show your partner (they don't have a manual either!). Therefore, an essential part of your dilation schedule is finding out what turns you on.

Positions

There is no right or wrong here.

A lot of women will find that positions that give them more control are best when starting. Girl on top is usually best for this. Have your partner relax and stay still, this way you can take him inside in your own time.

Lubrication and stimulation make for good sex and will help relax your pelvic floor.

If you have access to a Pelvic Physical Therapy Team, they can also offer practical advice and exercises to make this as awesome an experience as it should be.

Will I lubricate?

Lubricant is every girl's best friend when having sex. When cisgender females are surveyed **30**% ages 18 to 59 experienced difficulty with vaginal lubrication during the most recent time, they had sex. This is certainly not just a neo-vagina phenomenon!

It will make everything go a lot smoother. Some transgender women will certainly report being able to lubricate this may well be possible by the same mechanism that produces pre-ejaculate emissions or "pre-cum". This fluid comes from either the bulbourethral (Cowper's) glands and to a lesser extent by the

mucus-secreting urethral glands of Littre. Just like pre-ejaculate the amount of fluid produced is highly variable so just like you wouldn't dilate without lube do everyone a favor and have it around during sex.

Safe sex

Always remember to practice safe sex! This means your partner should wear a condom every time until you are both tested and only having sex with each other. Sexually transmitted diseases can be transmitted to your new vagina – protect it!

Douching

Because your vagina is lined with skin douching becomes an important part of taking care of it.

Just like the skin on the outside of your body needs to be cleaned with soap and water so does the inside.

At first when you are dilating often and leaving a lot of lubricant up there more frequent douching is required. You will not need to douche every time you dilate but you will want to clean up excess lubricant from your dilation sessions. Wiping the outside with a wet cloth is sufficient. Also, during healing some dead cells will fall off the lining and come out as a brown thick discharge.

Douching more frequently (see schedule below) will help with that.

Sample Douching Schedule

- o Week 1 and 2 after surgery douche daily

- o Week 3 and 4 after surgery douche every other day

- o After that 3 times a week (can be just done whenever you shower).

If you develop a lot of yellowish discharge or a bad odor your doctor may put you on a douching regimen with anti-bacterial solution. Alternatively, you may need a prescription antibiotic gel.

Urination

Welcome to the world of having a shorter urethra! When your surgeon does your surgery, they usually shorten the urethra by a few inches.

Therefore, it functions a little differently and can certainly take some getting used to.

1. Don't worry!

   Give it TIME after surgery when the catheter comes out (usually at about a week) things are still very swollen down there on the inside and outside. Accidents ARE COMMON. You may not make it to the bathroom on time (urge incontinence) or some leakage may happen when coughing or laughing stress incontinence). This will usually settle down.

2. Sitting to pee!

   In the first few months the urine stream is oftentimes unpredictable and may spray in inconvenient directions. The good news is this improves as will your sitting to pee technique! However, of note every girl at some point may have urine stream off onto the thigh when one of the labia gets in the way. Just another fun part of being a girl and toilet tissue will help.

3. What to watch out for

   If you are having uncomfortable symptoms such as burning or stinging when you pee. Lower belly pain or having to go a lot you may have an infection or "urinary tract infection". These are unfortunately very common as the urethra (tube from where the urine comes) is shorter and bacteria can easily get into the bladder. You are probably now at about the same risk as cis-gender females. Tricks to avoid it include always wiping from front to back and urinating after sex and dilation.

4. If you DO have a UTI

   Most primary care doctors will be comfortable treating a UTI in a transgender woman. However, it is very important for you to always remember that you do still have a prostate (a small one) but it also needs to be treated so this usually means some extra days (10-14 days) on antibiotics. Therefore, your doctor NEEDS to know your anatomy in order to treat you correctly.

Life after Vaginoplasty

Labiaplasty

Will I need a labiaplasty?

Labiaplasty is an umbrella term we use to talk about any other surgery or "nip- tuck" a patient may want to improve the appearance of her genitalia. Typically, this may be a scar revision, removal of lumps or bumps or making the outer lips meet in the middle. But it can include revision of the clitoris labia minora or vaginal opening. However, many of our patients may not ever want or need a labiaplasty once everything is healed.

When should I have it?

The golden rule with all secondary or revision surgeries is WAIT.

For 2 reasons

1. Your body will continue to improve on the appearance for about a year

2. Rushing back in, in the first few months after surgery is never a good idea and should be avoided as the anatomy is often "stuck together" as it heals leading to a possibly higher rate of complications.

We therefore prefer to wait a few months after the first surgery. Exceptions to this however are when the patient has a complication and may need a revision sooner to ensure everything continues to work smoothly.

What does labiaplasty involve?

For most patients this will be pretty quick outpatient procedure. Depending on how much work is done down time is usually a couple of days to a week.

4. Facial Surgery for Transfeminine Patients and Non-Binary Patients Assigned Male at Birth

Dr Barry Eppley

Introduction

The shape of the face has numerous features that give it a very gender specific appearance. Altering these facial features is an essential part of the changes needed for the male to female or female to male transgender patient. Facial feminization is by far more commonly done than facial masculinization in transgender surgery. This is likely due to the fact a softer male face is more socially acceptable than a stronger or harsher female face.

Facial reshaping surgery is very different than traditional facial rejuvenation surgery. Changing the structure of the face largely alters the natural bony framework which strongly contributes to its external appearance. Conversely facial rejuvenation surgery mainly changes the overlying soft tissues which have been adversely affected by aging. Conceptually facial feminization focuses on facial bone reduction while facial masculinization often involves facial bone augmentation.

Facial Feminization Surgery

Having a softer and more feminine face is the goal of facial feminization surgery. (FFS) While most commonly associated with the transgender patient, FFS is also used for the non-transgender female who feels their facial appearance is too masculine or has one facial feature that is considered excessively strong for their facial appearance.

Facial feminization surgery is a collection of reshaping procedures that can be done from the skull down to the neck. The three major facial thirds are analyzed, and a treatment plan is established for the maximal feminizing effect. Most FFS procedures involve bone reduction/reshaping although a few of the changes involve just soft tissue.

While some treatment centers offer a standard 'FFS package' it is important to realize that not every patient needs the exact same FFS surgery. And not every FFS procedure is done in a single surgery. But almost all FFS surgeries involve multiple facial procedures done at the same time.

Preoperative Evaluation

Since most of the facial changes done in FFS are largely either irreversible or difficult to reverse, it is critically important that the patient has the best knowledge as to what the impact of the proposed procedures will create. While any FFS procedure can be performed on a patient who seeks the surgery, the critical question is whether such changes will produce the desired aesthetic outcome. This speaks to the value of undergoing preoperative computer imaging to see the effects the selected facial changes may create. While computer imaging is an approximation of the surgeon's belief as to how the facial changes may appear after surgery, it provides an invaluable visual guide for the patient to determine both the value of the surgery and what facial procedures would work the best. No form of structural facial surgery should be done without a preoperative computer imaging evaluation.

Facial Feminization Surgery Procedures

Facial feminization surgery (FFS) is most common performed by board-certified plastic surgeons, all of which specialize in this type of facial surgery and many of whom have had craniofacial surgical training and experience. Surgery may be performed in an outpatient surgery center or a hospital depending upon what procedures are been done and whether the procedures may be covered by insurance. Time in surgery depends on the location and number of facial procedures being done. Surgery could be one hour or take up to 8 to 10 hours to perform. The facial procedures are always performed under general anesthesia (asleep). You can discuss the appropriate type of anesthesia with your doctor and the anesthesiologist. Some FFS procedures are done as an outpatient, but more extensive facial reshaping procedures will require an overnight stay.

FFS procedures are divided into four zones of treatment; skull/forehead, midface, lower jaw and neck.

FOREHEAD/SKULL
(Upper Third)

In this section the art of feminine reshaping of the upper third of the face will discuss the role of the following procedures:

1) Brow bone reduction

2) Tail of brow bone reduction

3) Vertical forehead length reduction

4) Bony forehead reshaping

5) Forehead augmentation

6) Brow lifting

7) Hair transplantation

Brow Bone Reduction (Central)

Considered one of the cornerstones of FFS surgery is the shape of the upper third of the face. Eliminating protruding brows and altering the appearance of the forehead to a more convex shape with a straighter vertical angulation is a critical gender difference between men and women. Always done through a superior incisional approach, the options are either the coronal (behind the frontal hairline) or pretrichial (at the frontal hairline) incision. This will be highly dependent on the location and hair density of the front hairline which is often not good in many male to female transgender patients. The pretichial incision offers more direct access to the brow bones and other forehead manipulations and is less traumatic to the hair. If hair transplantation is being considered to fill in or lower the frontal hairline the bony work should always be done first.

Reduction of the brow bones is most effectively done through a bone flap removal and replacement technique. While burring may be effective for a small number of patients, it cannot create the more significant brow bone reduction often needed due to the presence of the underlying frontal sinus. Taking the bone off over the front sinus, reshaping it and reducing the sinus perimeter edges, and then bone flap inset allows for a more significant central brow bone reduction. One critical area that is often overlooked is the frontonasal angle where the lower end of the bone meets the upper nasal bones. Ensuring that this one is deepened (lower radix height) is one of the defining measures of the success of the brow bone reduction procedure.

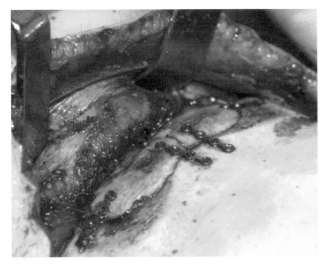

Figure 32 Microplate fixation of brow bone reduction

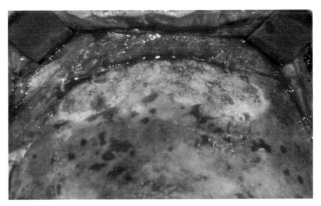

Figure 33 Maximal brow bone reduction with obliteration of the sinus using hydroxyapatite cement

In some secondary cases where the amount of desired brow bone reduction that has been achieved, maximal reduction can be assured by obliteration of the frontal sinus. The bone flap is used in a particular fashion instead of a bone graft for the frontonasal duct and the frontal sinus cavity obliterated with hydroxyapatite cement. This allows the central brow bone to be reduced as far back as needed. (extreme brow bone reduction)

Brow Bone Reduction (Lateral)

While much focus is often placed on the central brow bone area, not to be forgotten is the outer half of the supraorbital rims. (tail of the brow bones) Laying outside of the frontal sinus cavities the outer brows can be reshaped by burring to create a tail of the brow that has less projection and sweeps more upwardly which opens up the outer eye. This is a distinct female feature that helps soften the appearance of the forehead and when done with a temporal browlift can have a significant eyebrow reshaping effect. This should be part of most feminizing brow bone procedures and the bone in this area can be liberally reduced due to the lack of any underlying frontal sinus.

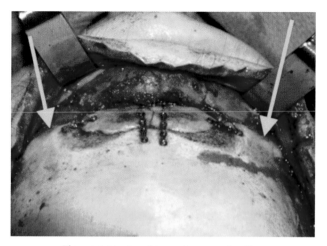

Figure 34 Lateral brow bone reduction

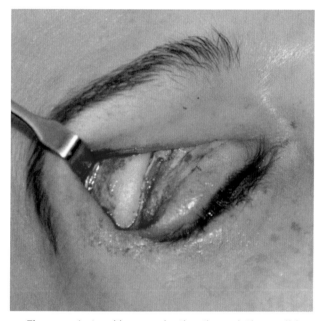

Figure 35 Lateral brow reduction through the eyelid

In patients who did not have the outer brow reshaped during their primary brow bone reduction or only need the tail of the brow bones treated, a more direct approach can be taken through an upper eyelid incision. It is not necessary to use a scalp or frontal hairline incisions to do so. This not only provides very direct access but also allows both horizontal and vertical bone reduction of the tail of the brow bone. It only requires a partial or lateral upper eyelid incision of which the scar outcome is similar to a traditional upper blepharoplasty for anti-aging effects.

Forehead Reduction (Soft Tissue)

A long or high forehead based on the location of the frontal hairline creates a disproportionately large upper third of the face. While acceptable in males because of common hairline recession/loss, it is much less aesthetic in females. Shortening of the upper facial third by frontal hairline advancement (scalp advancement) is one form of forehead reduction that is very common in the male to female conversion patient. How much the hairline can be advanced is dependent on the natural flexibility of one's scalp. (1.0 to 1.5cms) The most significant hairline advancements are created by a first stage scalp expansion procedure where the occipital scalp (not the scalp right behind the hairline) is treated by the placement of a tissue expander. Subsequent tissue expansions are done for 4 to 6 weeks prior to the definitive forehead procedure. This can permit up to 3 cms of hairline advancement to be achieved. Some hairlines, however, may not always permit this to be done due to a lack of hair density. But when possible a pretrichial incision permits a simultaneous brow bone and vertical skin forehead reduction to be accomplished.

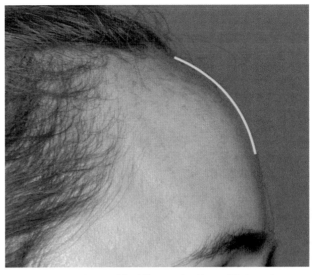

Figure 38 Frontal hairline reduction with bossing reduction before.

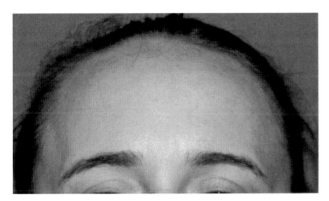

Figure 36 Fontal hairline advancement before

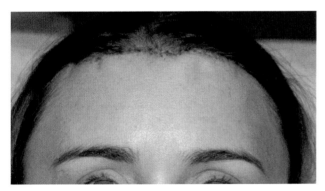

Figure 37 Frontal hairline advancement after

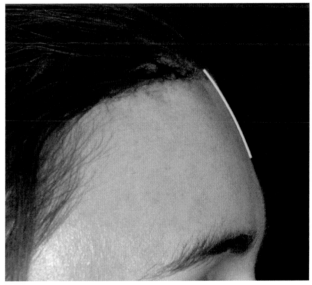

Figure 39 After

For some patients, even in those with only temporal hairline recession. hair transplantation can be a preferred choice. While taking more time to establish the definitive hairline than a frontal hairline advancement, it is more versatile and scar-less at the recipient site. hair transplantation is able to fill in temporal recessions and expand the anterior edge of the temporal hairline down towards the preauricular area, which a hairline advancement cannot do.

Bony Forehead Reduction

The other form of forehead reduction is to manage its bony shape above the brow bones. Frequently overlooked are the shapes of the central bony forehead and the lateral bony temporal lines. Some patients may have frontal bossing or a bowed out upper forehead area. While it is more common to build out the upper forehead to create a more feminine straight and convex forehead, there are patients where the bony projection of the upper forehead needs to be lessened to complement the brow bone reduction change. The thickness of the frontal bone will permit a 5 to 6mms reduction which will suffice in most patients to reduce any visible prominence.

Such bone shaving can be done to help create an increased convexity of the forehead shape by eliminating the visible ridge of the temporal lines. The temporal lines are the conversion area of the bony forehead to the soft tissue temporal muscle and fascia. In men this is more pronounced and burring it down helps create more of a side to side convex shape.

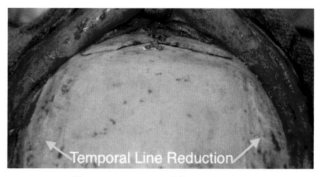
Figure 40 Temporal line reduction

Forehead Augmentation

In some patients with a flatter central forehead plateau, building it up with a small amount of bone cement (combined with temporal line reduction) is a dual approach to creating a more feminine forehead shape. The most common forehead cement to use is PMMA due to its favorable working properties and low cost. Hydroxyapatite cement (HA) is the synthetic equivalent to the mineral content of bone but costs considerably more to use.

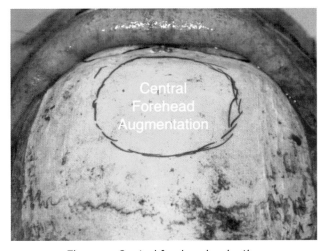

Figure 41 Central forehead reduction

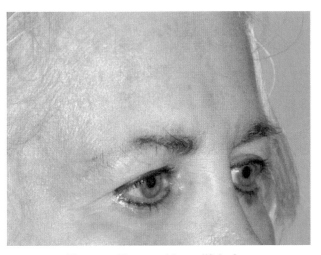

Figure 42 Temporal brow lift before

Browlift

While the brow bone projection can be reduced and the forehead reshaped, the appearance of the upper face may still not be fully feminized in some patients. The arch of the eyebrows has an important feminizing influence and a brow lift with any type of forehead surgery can have a substantial gender enhancing effect. Lifting the brows, particularly their tails, creates a distinct arch to the eyebrows which many females desire.

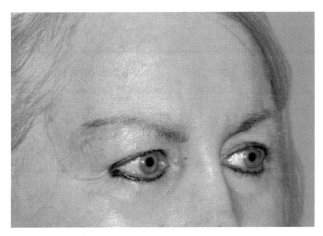

Figure 43 Temporal brow lift after

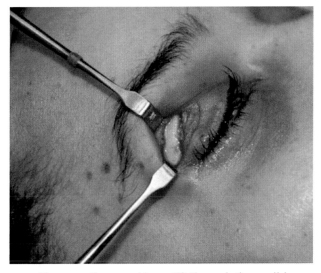

Figure 44 Temporal brow lift through the eyelid

Browlifting with Brow Bone Reduction/Forehead Reshaping

Browlifting can be concurrently done with any brow bone reduction either through a coronal scalp or pretrichial incisional approach. When done with brow bone reduction/forehead reshaping the most effective and controllable browlift technique is done with a pretrichial hairline incision. In this technique upper forehead skin can be removed to create the change in brow elevation directly below it. (inner two thirds of the brows) A tail of the brow elevation requires an incision either at the temporal hairline or behind it to create the necessary lifting effect. In lifting the tail of the brow, it is important to recognize that this portion of the brow must be lifted either equal to or often greater than the position of the inner half of the eyebrow. Many women prefer the upward sweep of the tail of the brow which is not a classically taught approach to traditional browlift surgery.

One of the 'problems' with the use of the coronal incision and brow lifting is that it works by removing a strip of scalp skin/hair to create its effect. While this is the original form of browlift surgery and has been used for decades (although largely not frequently today) the removal of a strip of scalp seems like a waste of good hair that may be in short supply for some patients.

Temporal Browlifts

Browlift surgery can be done as an independent procedure or secondarily after the bony work of the forehead/brow bones, either as a known preoperative decision or to complement the previous work. What approach to use depends on the brow reshaping effect desired? Most of the time in the transgender FFS patient the focus is on the tail of the brow area and getting that upward temporal sweep of the arch. The best method to do so is the combined transpalpebral-temporal incisional technique. By coming from below through the upper eyelid complete undermining and maximal mobilization of the tail of the brow can be achieved. This also creates the opportunity to do any tail of the brow bone reduction by burring if desired. Through a small temporal incision behind the hairline the tail of the brow can be resuspended by sutures to the deep temporal fascia way behind the incision.

Some females desire an 'extreme' or Cat Eye type of change to the outer eye/brow area. Like all maximal procedures it requires a maximal effort. This requires a combination of a transpalpebral-temporal tail of the browlift, with or without brow bone reduction, with a lateral canthoplasty to effect a change in position of the corner of the eye as well.

Skull Reduction/Reshaping

While the forehead has some prominent gender differences, the shape of the rest of the skull is less significant in that regard. But differences do exist, and the general trend is that male head shapes are larger and broader while female head shapes are a little smaller and more round. The camouflage of hair can make these differences irrelevant for many women but not for all. Skull reductions are not rare in male to female transgender patients. The typically reduced areas include a wider side of the head and a more prominent bony temporal line as it extends back from the forehead to the back of the head at the parietal bone.

Bony reduction of the prominent temporal lines or from side to side to reduce vertical skull height as well is done by removing the outer cortical bone layer down to the diploic space. This is in the range of 5 to 7mms depending on the skull's thickness. Some form of superior scalp incision is needed but not to the extent of a full coronal type incision.

Reducing the wide side of the head is typically done by posterior temporal muscle removal from an incision behind the ear. While many think that this requires bone removal the muscle actually makes a bigger contribution to head width and is more easily removed. While the bone also can be reduced by burring this is not usually necessary and requires extending the incision from behind the ear further up along the side of the head. Removing the portion of the temporal muscle has no adverse effects on mouth opening and closing.

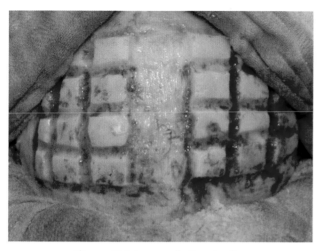

Figure 45 Intra-op skull reduction

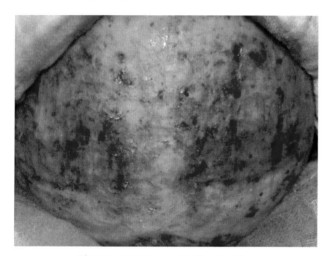

Figure 46 Intra-op skull reduction

MIDFACE *(Middle Third)*

In this section the art of feminine reshaping of the middle third of the face will discuss the role of the following procedures:

1) Rhinoplasty

2) Cheek Augmentation

3) Buccal Lipectomies and Perioral Liposuction

4) Eye Corner Lifting

5) Infraorbital Augmentation

6) Earlobe Reduction

7) Ear Reduction

Rhinoplasty

There are major gender differences in the shape of the nose. In achieving a more feminine-looking nose the key is the shape of the dorsum (bridge) and the tip. A straight or preferably slightly concave dorsum with a tip that is narrow and with a nasolabial angle that is more open and of at least 110 degrees is preferred. Lowering the central dorsum to create a slight saddle appearance and having a significant tip rotation, and tip deprojection if necessary, has a very feminizing effect. Good tip rotation is important but should not be done so much that excessive nostril show occurs. Getting the radix of the nose lowered (height of the nose between the eyes) is a key feature and is best achieved when done at the same time as a brow bone reduction. (as coming from above is the easiest and most assured method of lowering it)

To some degree feminizing a nose potentially violates adequate support for the middle third of the nose and potential nasal airway compromise. But this can be avoided by adequate cartilage graft support.

An open rhinoplasty is usually needed to reliably achieve these nose shape changes. Because in most male to female rhinoplasties it is a reductive operation extensive cartilage grafting is not needed. But septal cartilage grafts for the columella and possible the middle vault are commonly used.

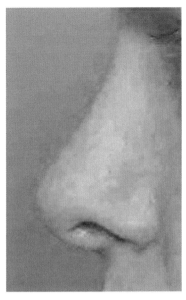
Figure 48 Feminizing rhinoplasty after

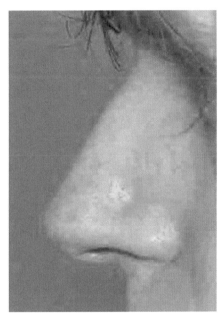
Figure 47 Feminizing rhinoplasty before

Cheek Augmentation

Feminine cheeks typically have more fullness in the 'apple' cheek area, which is on the front part of the cheekbone, the malar-submalar zone. This aesthetic female cheek roundness is historic, although more contemporary trends for cheek augmentation are for a line of fullness that extends back along the zygomatic arch as well for more defined and linear cheek highlights. The desired cheek augmentation look will help define the best method to achieve it.

The most common non-surgical method for cheek augmentation is done with the use of injectable fillers. A wide variety of injectable fillers now exist and more highly cross-linked hyaluronic-acid fillers (e.g., Voluma) work well in the cheeks. Longer-lasting effects can come from Sculptra although multiple treatments are needed to achieve the optimal effect. While these are effective they are not permanent which on the surface seems unfavorable. But more permanent injectable fillers should be approached with caution. Should an inflammatory response develop, or lumps/irregularities occur months to years later, they can be more difficult problems to solve.

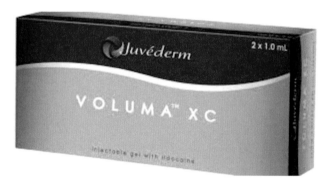

Figure 49 Juvaderm filler

Fat injections are a surgical technique for cheek augmentation that is appropriate to consider when one is already having other surgeries. Using one's own fat is a 'natural' approach that has its best track record of survival in the cheeks. Fat injections can be very effective for the softer look of a cheek augmentation.

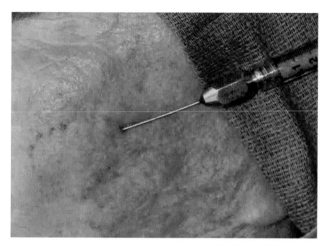

Figure 50 Cheek augmentation with fat grafting

Permanent cheek augmentation can be done using either standard or custom cheek implants. Several different styles of standard cheek implants exist for the malar, submalar and combined malar-submalar cheek areas. The combined malar-submalar implant, known as the malar shell implant, is most commonly used for its more complete volumizing effect. If one desires a higher cheek look with augmentation that extends back along the zygomatic arch a custom cheek implant design is used. With either type of cheek implant an intraoral approach is used for placement.

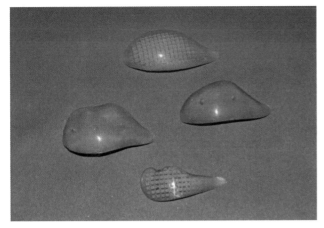

Figure 51 Standard cheek implant styles

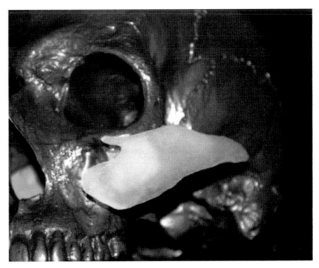

Figure 52 Female cheek implant design

An autologous or natural type of cheek augmentation can also be done by moving the cheekbone outward in a procedure known as a Zygomatic Sandwich Osteotomy. (ZSO) Through an intraoral approach an oblique osteotomy is done through the zygomatic body of the cheekbone. The cheekbone is moved outward and fixed with a plate and screws with or without an allogeneic bone graft. This type of cheekbone osteotomy creates lateral cheek fullness in the front part of the cheek.

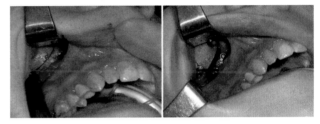

Figure 53 Zygoma sandwich osteotomy technique

Another cheek enhancing procedure is that of dimpleplasty. Cheek dimples can be created through an intraoral technique. Cheek dimples occur naturally because of a defect in the zygomaticus major muscle. This can be created by making a defect in the intraoral mucosa up to the underside of the skin in the desired dimple location. By suturing the underside of the skin down into the defect a dimple is created. Dimples occur only when smiling (dynamic dimples) or exist at rest and get deeper when smiling. (static dimples) The surgical techniques are slightly different to create either one.

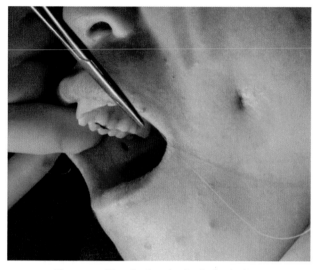

Figure 54 Cheek dimpleplasty technique

Buccal Lipectomies and Perioral Mound Liposuction

While not a classic feminizing procedure, midfacial defatting can be a useful facial reshaping technique for those patients who have naturally rounder faces or chubby cheeks. The three facial areas that can be successfully reduced by different techniques are the two primary cheek areas, the buccal fat pads and the perioral mounds, as well as that of the neck. Often all three are combined to maximize the amount of facial slimming that can be achieved.

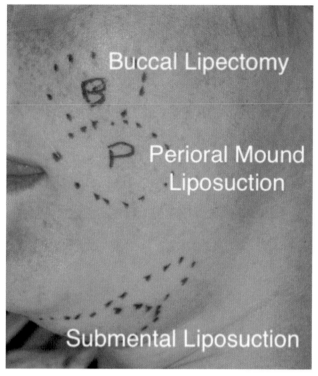

Figure 55 Liposuction areas

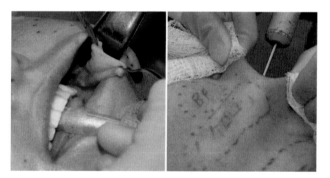

Figure 56 Facial lipectomy

The buccal fat pad is a relatively large collection of concentrated fat that sits right below the cheekbone that is easily accessed from a small intraoral incision in the cheek opposite the maxillary second molar. Its removal, either partially or totally, helps reduce upper cheek fullness. But it is important to know that its effects do not extend all the way down to the level of the mouth or the jawline. There is a common misconception that it does. For this reason perioral liposuction is a good complement to buccal lipectomies. This reduction in the thickness of the subcutaneous fat layer by the side of the mouth and down to the jawline creates a more complete cheek slimming effect. Done with a very small cannula from an incision just inside the corner of the mouth, this lower cheek area can be treated from the buccal fat area down to the jawline. This is a perfectly safe area to treat by liposuction due to the lack of any motor nerves that run in this area.

The dual effects of buccal lipectomies and perioral liposuction can create a noticeable slimming effect even in patients that don't really have a round or fuller facial shape. In the right face these defatting procedures can make the cheekbones look more prominent. In combination with even smaller cheek implants, a substantially enhanced cheekbone definition can be achieved.

Eye Corner Lifting

Feminizing the eye shape by contemporary standards is to elevate the outer corner of the eye. This elevation specifically refers to having the outer eye corner higher than the inner eye corner. At the least this alleviates a tired looking eye but females generally prefer a slight upturned outer eye corner. To reposition the outer eye corner higher a lateral canthoplasty technique is needed, not a lateral canthopexy. The lateral canthal tendons need to be released and moved up higher inside the lateral orbital rim. The most secure method of doing so is with transosseous holes for the suture fixation of the tendon to the bone. This is most conveniently done during a brow bone reduction or can be done independently using a small lateral upper eyelid incision. Emphasis is placed on elevating the outer eye corner for over correction as some settling will always occur.

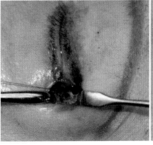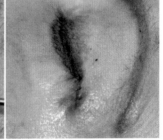

Figure 57 Lateral canthoplasty for eye reshaping

In its most exaggerated form, sometimes called *Cat Eye* surgery, the outer eye corner is significantly elevated which is often combined with a brow lift. This creates a complete upward temporal sweep look to the outer eye area.

Infraorbital Augmentation

While not necessarily a gender feature, hollowing under the eyes is an undesired midfacial appearance. (infraorbital hollowing) Given its location under the eye it is not going to be improved by any effect of cheek augmentation. (unless a custom infraorbital-malar implant is used) Like cheek augmentation, treatment options include injectable fillers, fat injections and implants with the same advantages and disadvantages for each one of them. The difference in the infraorbital area from that of the cheeks is that the overlying soft tissues are thinner and contour irregularities are much more common with fillers and fat. In addition the removal of any filling material (semi-permanent fillers and fat) may be less problematic than that of the cheeks but still requires an open lower blepharoplasty to do so.. For these reasons hyaluronic-based synthetic fillers or infraorbital implants are often better treatments and more easily

reversed. The options in permanent implants include standard tear trough and custom-made infraorbital implants.

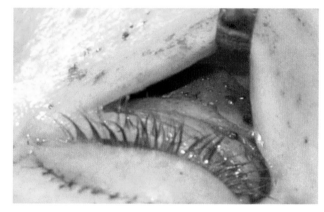

Figure 58 Tear trough implant

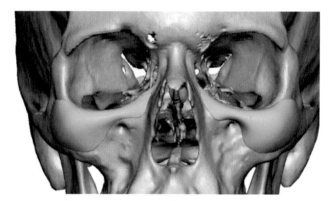

Figure 59 Custom infraorbital implants

Earlobe Reduction

The ears appear in the midface section because that is where they lie horizontally in alignment to the face.

Large earlobes are often tolerated on men but are less attractive and proportionate in women. While cisgenderb women often develop elongation of the only non-cartilaginous portion of the ear from ear ring wear and aging, a male to female patient may have them from natural development. Either way there are two techniques for earlobe reduction that are very effective and have well-hidden scars. The technique not to use is the classic wedge reduction through the middle of the earlobe where a resultant fine line scar ends up on its anterior surface. Depending upon the natural attachment of the earlobe to the side of the face (attached vs unattached) reduction can be done using an inferior helical rim excision (unattached earlobe) or wedge excision at the attachment of the earlobe the face. (attached earlobe)

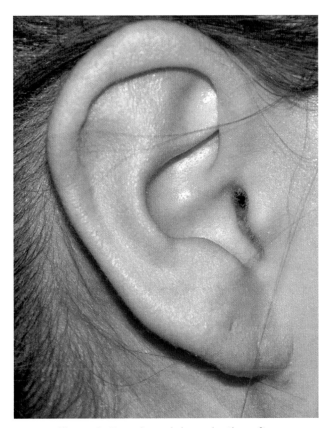

Figure 61 Female earlobe reduction after

Ear Reduction

The female ear is typically smaller in size/height than that of men. In some patients a large ear may be due to just enlargement of the lower earlobe which can be reduced as previously discussed. But when the ear is large due to being vertically long in height, which may or may not be associated with a large earlobe in the lower third, the typical cause is an enlarged upper third. This is from an enlarged scaphal cartilage segment. Vertical ear reduction or macrotia reduction surgery is done by removal of outer

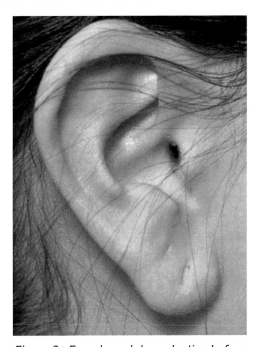

Figure 60 Female earlobe reduction before

skin and cartilage from the scapha and a designated section of helical rim cartilage and skin. This allows a downward rotation of a helical rim flap. This lowers the height of the upper third of the ear and keeps the scar line inside the helical rim...with the exception of a very small fine line across the mid portion of the helical rim. Int many cases of large ears the earlobe is also reduced with an inferior helical rim excision. Either of these 'high and low' approaches create a visible reduction in the size of the ear. Vertical ear reductions are typically in the range of 10 to15mms.

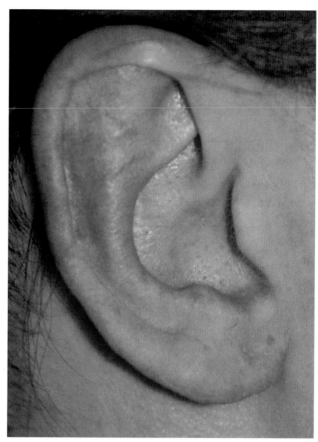

Figure 63 Vertical ear reduction after

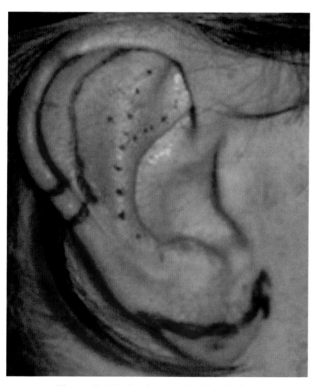

Figure 62 Vertical ear reduction before

LOWER FACE (Lower Third)

In this section the art of feminine reshaping of the lower third of the face, we will discuss the role of the following procedures:

1) Perioral Enhancements

2) Chin Reduction

3) Masseter Muscle Reduction

4) Jaw Angle Reduction

5) V-Line Jaw Reduction

6) Tracheal Shave

7) Neck Liposuction

8) Submentoplasty

9) Lower Facelift

Perioral Enhancements

Lip Injections

Enhancing the shape and size of the upper and lower lips can be one of the most powerful gender facial changes. Though small in size their impact on gender identification is significant. A variety of surgical and non-surgical lip augmentation procedures exist. The most common form of lip augmentation done is with the use of injectable fillers. Besides being temporary its effectiveness is based on having enough vertical vermilion height to allow a visible volume increase without having excess horizontal protrusion. (duck appearance) Fat injections can also be used but they have such a poor history of successful survival in the lips that they are the least used method for lip augmentation.

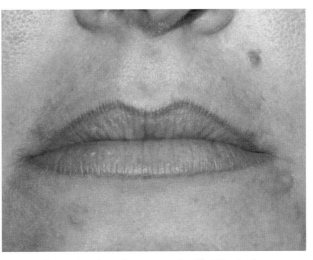

Figure 64 Lip enhancement with filler before

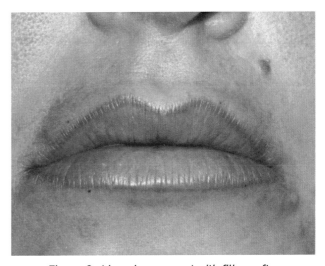

Figure 65 Lip enhancement with fillers after

Lip Implants

This same issue applies to lip implants where their effectiveness is dependent on having adequate vermilion and a good Cupid's bow shape initially. To convert the male lip to a more feminine appearance, surgical lip augmentation methods can be more effective and permanent.

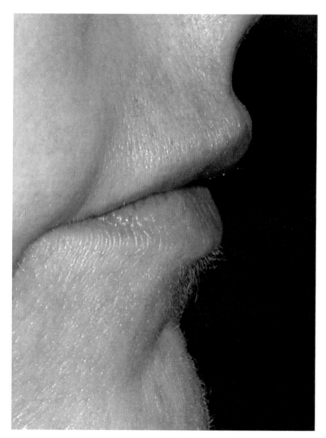

Figure 66 Upper lip implant before side view

Subnasal Lip Lifts

There are four surgical lip augmentation procedures available; subnasal lip lifts, vermilion advancements, V-Y mucosal advancements and corner of mouth lifts. When the vertical distance between the base of the nose and the upper lip is long (which many men have) and the sides of the upper lip vermilion have adequate height, the subnasal lip lift is ideal. By removing skin from under the nose the upper lip skin distance is shortened and the Cupid bow area looks fuller and more upturned.

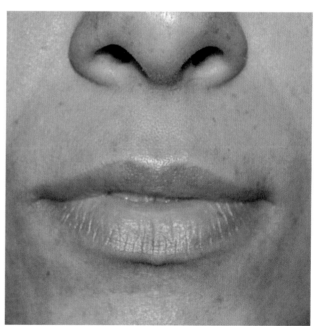

Figure 68 Sub-nasal lip lift before

Figure 67 Upper lip implant after

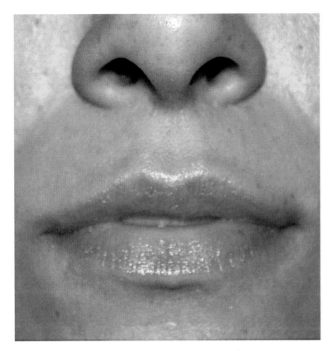

Figure 69 Sub-nasal lip lift after

Lip Advancements

When the upper lip is very thin from corner to corner the preferred procedure is a vermilion or upper lip advancement. Lip advancements change the location and shape of the vermilion border and create the most powerful and permanent method to enhance the size of a once thin male upper lip. It is the only procedure that can make a more pronounced Cupid's bow when it doesn't exist. The very fine line scar along the vermilion-skin border heals very well. It can also be equally applied to the lower lip. When vermilion advancements are done in both the upper and lower

lip concurrently the mouth area is dramatically feminized.

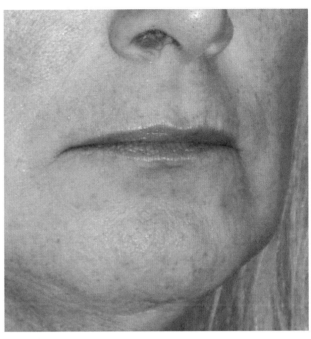

Figure 70 Lip advancement before

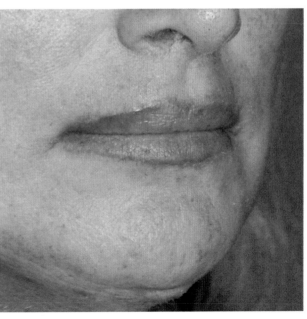

Figure 71 Lip advancement after

V-Y Mucosal Advancements

Another less frequently used method of lip augmentation is an internal approach the leaves no external scars lines. By rolling out the internal wet mucosa of the lip in a specific V-Y form of advancement, the underside of the lip is more exposed making the lips bigger. This only really works well of the patient already has an adequate amount of dry vermilion height.

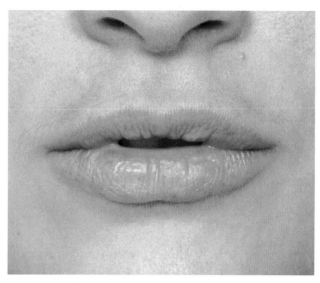

Figure 72 V-Y advancement before

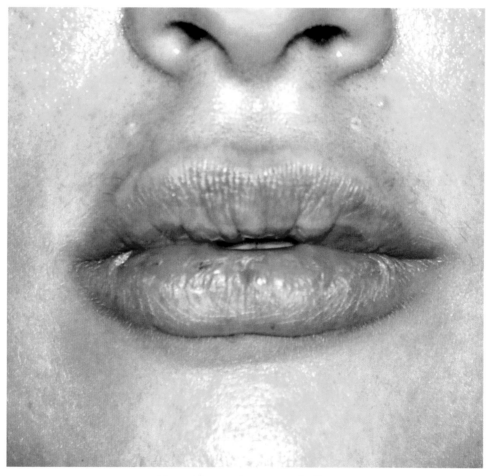

Figure 73 v-y advancement after

Corner of Mouth Lifts

Downturned or dropping corners of the mouth, in any gender, does not offer a pleasing appearance. The most effective and permanent procedure is a corner of the mouth lift. The historic method for doing so leaves unfavorable scars beyond the vermilion-skin junction and has been replaced with a pennant excision technique. This allows the mouth corner vermilion to be placed more level or upturned while keeping the fine scar line at the preferred skin-vermilion edge around the entire corner of the mouth.

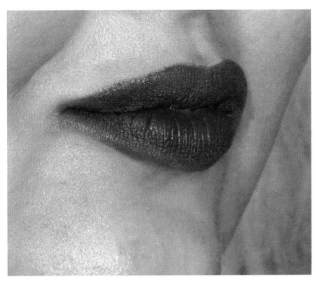

Figure 75 Corner of the mouth lift after

Chin Reduction

Chin Narrowing

A large or prominent chin is a distinct male feature and is one of the most important changes to make for a more feminine lower face. In determining the type of chin reduction procedure needed it is important to determine the dimensional changes required for the desired effect. In some chin shapes the horizontal projection and vertical length are fine but the chin is too wide. For this chin shape change the corners of the chin are removed with a reciprocating saw through an intraoral approach (lateral tubercle reduction). This is the one chin reduction procedure where bone burring from an intraoral approach can be effective.

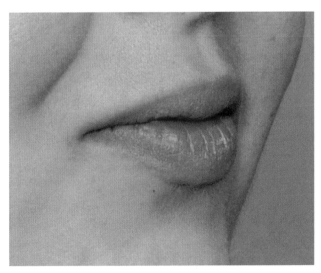

Figure 74 Corner of mouth lift before

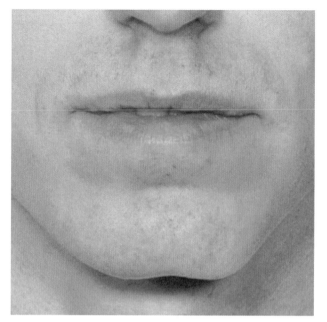

Figure 76 Chin narrowing via intra-oral approach before

where horizontal and vertical sections of bone are removed, and the chin reassembled with small plates and screws. If a horizontal deficiency chin exists as well, the reassembled chin bones can be made to add increased horizontal projection. This can be a very favorable change for the patient seeking a more tapered chin shape from the frontal view.

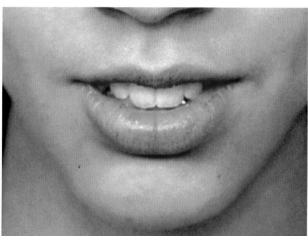

Figure 78 Chin narrowing via sliding genioplasty before

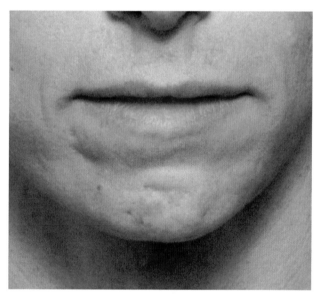

Figure 77 Chin narrowing via intra-oral approach after

Chin Length and Width Reduction

Often, however, more than one dimension of the chin needs to be changed. To reduce the vertically long and wide chin, an intraoral t-shaped genioplasty is performed

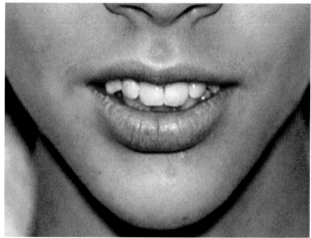

Figure 79 Chin narrowing by sliding genioplasty after

Chin Projection Reduction

The most challenging chin reduction to perform is when it is vertically long, wide and sticks out too far. (too much horizontal projection) Getting adequate horizontal reduction of the chin, along with the other dimensions must take into account what will happen to the soon to be excessive soft tissue chin pad. Only one chin reduction approach can satisfactorily reduce all three dimensions of the chin bone and remove the excess soft tissue as well...the external submental approach where a soft tissue excision and chin tuck can be performed at the same time.

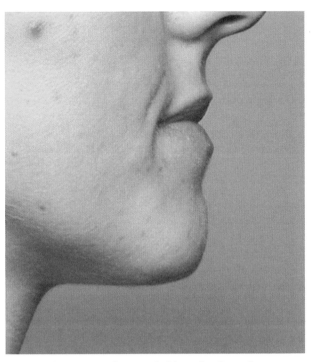

Figure 81 Submental chin reduction after

Jaw Reduction

Jaw reduction is a generic term for different types of lower facial reshaping procedures. Often lumped into one general category, the reality is that a variety of bone and muscle reduction procedures are available to create a lower face that appears more narrow or slimmer. Each jaw reduction procedure differs in the specific dimensional changes that are created in the lower face. The two general types of jaw reductions can target either muscle or bone.

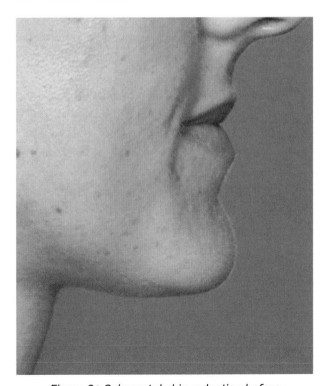

Figure 80 Submental chin reduction before

Masseter Muscle Reduction

The masseter muscle is a large soft tissue structure that is stretched out between the zygomatic arch (origin) and the bony jaw angle (insertion). When the masseter muscle is overly enlarged due to natural congenital size, or hypertrophied due to over activity (e.g., chronic clenching) it can create a wide looking lower jaw. It can be treated non-surgically by Botox injections. (or Dysport or Xeomin) This works by causing a reduction in the size of the muscle fibers which reduces the thickness of the muscle. Th injections are localized to the part of the muscle over the bony jaw angle below the ear which is coincidentally the safest place for injection therapy to avoid buccal branches of the facial nerve which lie above it. The effect of the muscle reduction is usually seen by about three weeks after an injection treatment and will last about 3 months when the size of the muscle slowly returns. In some patients with enough Botox treatments the reduction in the size of the masseter muscles may be longer lasting or even permanent but this is the exception and does not commonly occur.

Surgical masseter muscle reduction can also be done but this does not refer to the excision of segments of the muscle. This is generally not a preferred technique of muscle reduction due to the risks of intraoperative bleeding and the high likelihood of creating external contour irregularities. An alternative approach which is similar to radiofrequency ablation is electocautery reduction. With this technique an incision is made inside the mouth and the inner surface of the muscle is lifted off of the bone. The inner surface of the muscle is then treated by direct electrocautery using a fine tipped needle at spot locations in a grid pattern. This has no risks of causing bleeding or muscle irregularities. The thermal injury to the muscle cause it to partially shrink over time, this reduction will be permanent due to loss of muscle fibers.

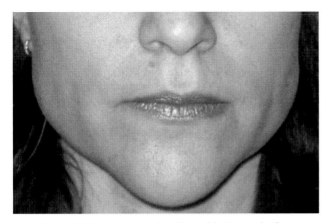

Figure 82 Masseter reduction with Botox before

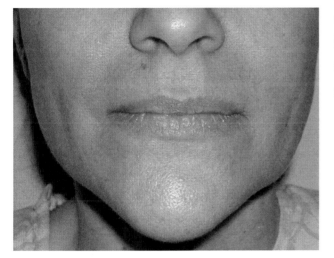

Figure 83 Masseter reduction with Botox after

Bony Jaw Reduction

Jaw Angle Reduction

While the chin is the leading corner of the lower jaw, the jaw angles are the paired back corners. Like the chin they can be similarly reduced although their dimensional changes are less complex when done in isolation. Reducing their width or flare makes the appearance of the jawline slimmer from the front view and creates a facial shape less wide or square. By reducing their width but not the vertical length the shape of the jaw angle is preserved and there is little risk of soft tissue sag due to loss of bony support. This is typically done through an intraoral approach by a bone burring technique to remove the outer layer of bone and jaw angle point. It can also be done more directly from an external skin incision in the neck if one wants to completely avoid the recovery from an intraoral approach.

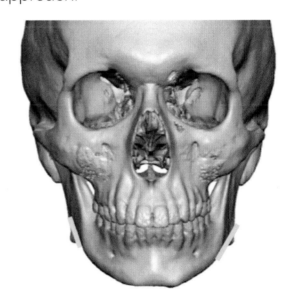

Figure 84 Jaw angle reduction

V Line Jaw Reduction

The term 'v line surgery' refers to a complete or total jaw reduction procedure, that reduces the bone from the jaw angles in the back to the chin in the front. It can be a confusing term because it technically has several variations, which differ based on the specific dimensions of the jaw that need to be reduced. Jawbone removal can be done either in a partial thickness (shaving or lateral corticotomies) or full thickness excision. (ostectomies)

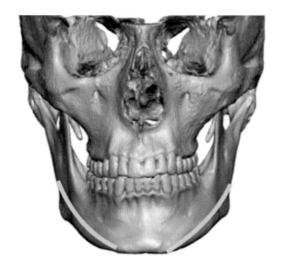

Figure 85 V line jaw reduction

For patients with very wide and/or a vertically long lower jaw, a full thickness of bone is removed in a curved fashion from the jaw angles to the chin. This changes the complete shape of the bone not only in width but in length as well (changes the mandibular plane angle). It produces the most dramatic amount of jaw reduction but also risks over-resection when applied to the wrong type of jaw shape. This is what is done in traditional v-line surgery. It is no surprise that this type of jaw reduction emanates from Asia where the natural shape of the lower jaw is more square and needs full thickness excisions for a significant shape change and a more noticeable narrowing effect.

While less well-known V line surgery can also be done by shaving or by removing the outer layer of bone which changes the width of the jaw but not its vertical length. The jaw angle shape is kept intact but it becomes less wide. The amount of jaw reduction change is less dramatic but is more aesthetically appropriate for jaw shapes that are not unduly wide or flared and don't have a low jaw angle. It is often better suited to the patient who has a normal mandibular plane angle and has little risk of resulting in an over resected lower jaw shape.

The key to a successful bony jaw reduction is to match the technique with the dimensional requirements needed for the desired change. This not only requires preoperative x-rays (panorex, lateral cephalogram or 3D jaw CT scan) but computer imaging to determine what magnitude of jaw reduction change the patient desires. While under- and over resection results can occur, by far the most common revisional jaw reduction patients I see is when too much has been done. This almost always is when traditional v-line surgery has left the patient with over resected jaw angles and chin that is too narrow or elongated. This can be a function of overly aggressive bone reduction but more commonly occurs because it was not the right technique for the patient's natural jaw shape.

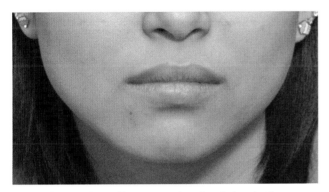

Figure 86 Jawline narrowing front view before

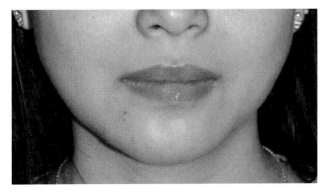

Figure 87 Jawline narrowing after

NECK

Tracheal Shave

A prominent Adam's apple or thyroid cartilage disrupts the profile of the neck and is the one sure sign of being male. It is reduced by a procedure that truly reflects how it is done... the tracheal shave. The prominent union of the two halves of the thyroid cartilage is shaved down through either a direct skin incision over it or from a more 'hidden' skin incision up under the chin. In younger patients the cartilage is soft and is readily modified by a scalpel blade in a shaving technique. In older patients, however, the thyroid cartilage will be firmer or calcified and a burring technique may be needed to achieve an adequate reduction of its prominence. While it is the 'simplest' of all FFS procedures it also incredibly effective in making the neck look more feminine without a visible bump, or a greatly reduced bump, as seen in profile.

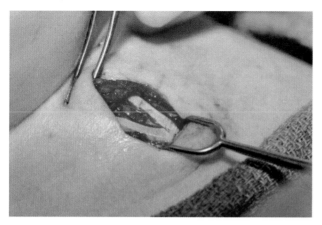

Figure 88 Tracheal shave intra-op

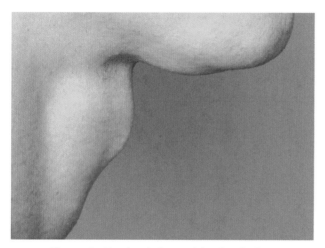

Figure 89 Tracheal shave side-view before

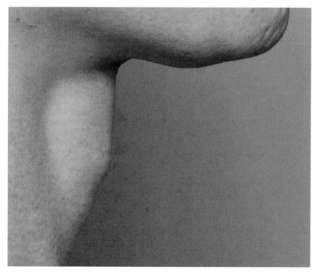

Figure 90 Tracheal shave side view after

Liposuction/Submentoplasty

An improved shape of the neck, due to excess fat can be achieved with small cannula liposuction. By reducing the subcutaneous layer of fat thickness between the skin and the platysma muscle, the overlying skin contracts down (upward) to show a more obvious cervicomental angle. This classic neck reshaping procedure is a good complement to chin and jawline changes.

In some patient's subcutaneous fat removal alone does not produce the ideal central cervicomental angle show. Fat removal below the platysma muscle centrally and tightening the two sides of the platysma muscle across it produces a more evident cervicomental angle as the neck is pulled up and back. This more complete central neck reshaping procedure is known as a submentoplasty or 'neck liposuction plus'.

Lower Facelift

In older FFS patients there may be laxity of the soft tissue along the jawline as well as in the neck. While a lower facelift may not be considered a classic FFS procedure, many older patients benefit by this jawline-neck reshaping procedure. It is both a rejuvenating and feminizing procedure with an improved sweep up along the jawline up into the ear area. Like all facelift surgery there are different magnitudes or levels of the surgery based on the severity of neck sagging and jowling. They can fundamentally be divided into level 1 (mini facelift with no neck work), level 2 (facelift with limited neck work (liposuction) and level 3 (full facelift with submentoplasty neck work). The extent of the facelift surgery is correlated to the magnitude of the aging process.

Facial Feminization Surgery Recovery

Recovery from any form of facial surgery is primarily related to how much swelling occurs and how long it takes to go away. Thus, recovery is more appearance-related than it is of functional limitations. This recovery period will be highly influenced by the number of FFS procedures that are performed. While there are some patients who only have one or two procedures that take a few hours of surgery, it is also not uncommon that multiple facial procedures are done

that can involve six to eight hours of surgery.

As a general guideline 50% of the facial swelling subsides by 10 to 14 days after surgery, two-thirds is gone by three weeks after surgery and it takes up to six weeks before most of the swelling is fully gone. It takes longer for the facial swelling and whatever bruising may occur to resolve than most patients realize although, the FFS patient seems to be more aware of this longer recovery time, than many other types of facial surgery patients. These are no physical restrictions after surgery and one can shower and wash their hair within 48 hours and every day thereafter. But when one feels comfortable being out in public or returning to work after surgery depends on how one feels about their facial appearance. The results of any facial surgery cannot be fully assessed until 3 months or so after the surgery when both the swelling has subsided, and the overlying soft tissues have contracted back down. Despite this somewhat long recovery period, most FFS patients can see some of the positive changes early on in the recovery period.

Complications and Risks

The potential complications from FFS surgery can be divided into medical and aesthetic risks. The most significant medical risks are that of infection, scars and permanent numbness of the sensory nerves around the operative sites. Any motor nerve weakness is rare although not an impossibility. These medical risks are, fortunately, not very common. Even the infection risk in the face and skull is very low due to its superb blood supply.

The aesthetic risks of FFS surgery are more common and are fundamentally about how the facial appearance has turned out in terms of degree of change, symmetry and smoothness of the results. There is always some risk of the need for revision of the procedures to optimize their aesthetic outcomes. As a general guideline it is wise to assume that any single operation has a 15% need for aesthetic revision. As multiple procedures are combined, as is common in FFS surgery, this risk is additive.... meaning that each procedure cumulatively adds to the risk. It is fair to assume that in a multiple procedure FFS surgery some revision surgery will almost always be needed.

Facial Feminization Surgery Cost

Costs for FFS surgery vary widely and depend on the number of procedures being done and the operative time it takes to do them. Each treatment plan is individualized from which the cost of surgery is determined after a consultation is completed. Such evaluations today can be done by a virtual consultation process based on photo analysis and computer imaging.

In some cases, FFS surgery may be covered by insurance. This is determined by a preoperative insurance predetermination process, a written submission by the plastic surgeon which contains all pertinent information for the insurance company to evaluate and make a coverage decision. While more insurance companies are providing coverage for transgender procedures than ever before, some still don't and not every FFS surgeon participates in insurance programs.

Consult a Qualified FFS Surgeon

Here are some tips to consider when consulting a surgeon about FFS:

- Create a list of the facial changes you think would be most helpful for the best transformation to discuss with your surgeon. This will help the surgeon understand your expectations and develop a treatment plan.

- Ask where the surgery will be performed, the extent of the procedure and whether it is going to be done as an outpatient or overnight stay.

- Ask about complications and possible side effects of the procedure. (they can and do happen)

- Ask the recovery period and your activities after surgery so you can plan properly for the time needed.

5. Top Surgery for the Transfeminine and Assigned Male at Birth Nonbinary Patient

Dr Sidhbh Gallagher

Feminizing Mastoplasty- Breast Augmentation and Breast lifts

Breast growth with hormones can be unpredictable. There is a belief that after the full effects a patient can expect to be one to two cup sizes smaller than her female relatives. In examining and talking to patients I don't find this to be necessarily true. There is also a lot of controversy as to what hormones create the best breasts. It is unclear if using estrogen and or progestins make a difference.

It does take time however for the hormones to take effect. Most doctors agree that it will take about 24 months after starting feminizing hormones to get the full effect.

For this reason, I strongly advise patients to wait and see what growth they get naturally and if your insurance company is going to cover the surgery, they will also often want documentation of 1-2 years of hormone therapy first.

Many transgender women notice that their breast may not have an ideal shape after breast growth. Often times what they complain of is a tuberous appearance to the breasts whereby the lower half of the breast does not round out nicely and the fold under the breast can be too high. In order to correct this a breast lift may also be required to reshape the breast – this is often called a feminizing mastoplasty.

The downside of this is that in order to effectively reshape the breast often scars are needed on the breast but in most patients, these will fade very well in time.

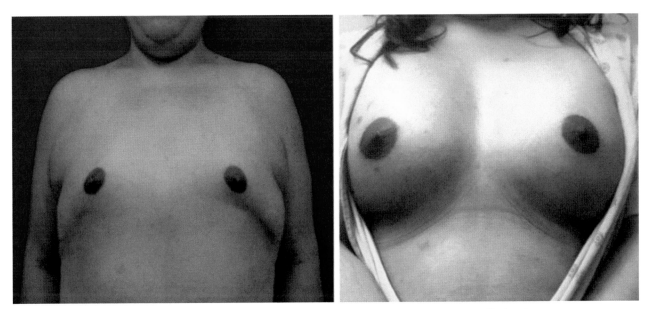

Figure 91 Front view of a transfeminine patient who had 800cc high profile implants placed in a subglandualar position.

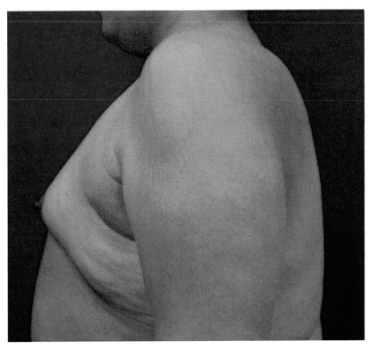

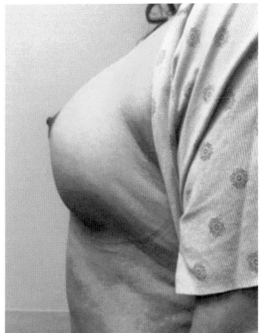

Figure 92 Side View

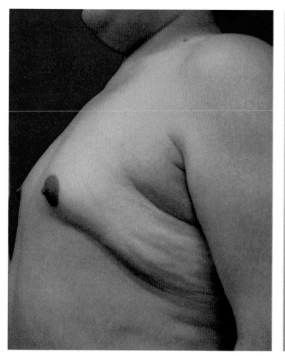
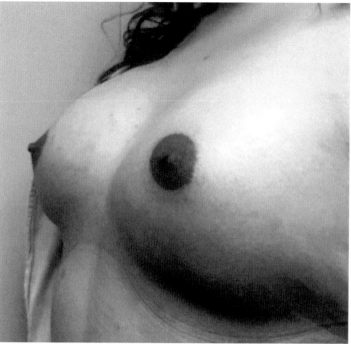

Figure 93 The scar was placed in the fold under the breast.

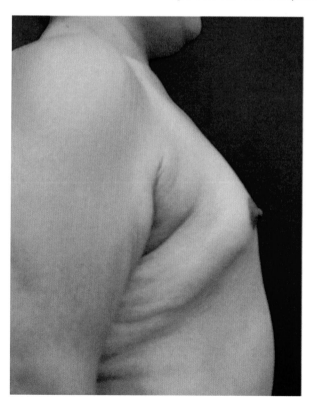
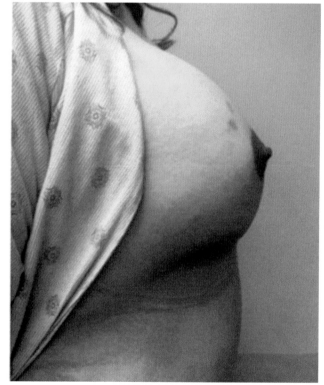

Figure 94 Side view

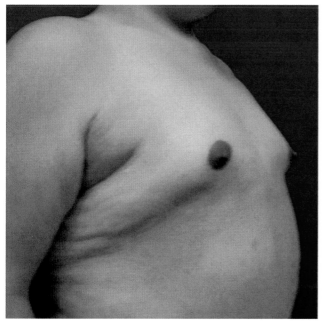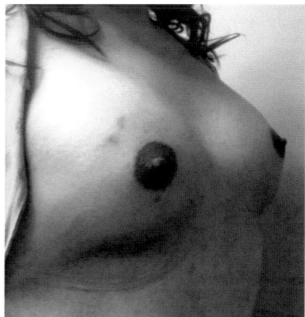

Figure 95 Three- quarter view

Breast Augmentation

This can be a wonderfully affirming procedure where the transgender woman will leave the hospital with the full look she has always hoped for. There are of course a couple of caveats with this procedure. It has limitations. Breast augmentation cannot completely reshape the chest.

Small areola will still be small, and the biggest complaint is usually the lack of cleavage in widely spaced breasts. This can be very tricky to get much of an improvement on. Uneven breasts may still be uneven despite the surgeon's best efforts. To know what she is signing up for I often ask patients to take a long look at their breasts in the mirror before surgery and note things they don't like about their appearance. In some cases, after the implants are placed these features can seem exaggerated (everything is bigger!). Those small areolae can now look tiny and the space between the breasts even larger.

Breast augmentation is not a miracle it is critical to understand what it can and can't do to feminize the chest.

Fat Grafting for Breast Augmentation

Although its less commonly done, it's important to note that a patient's breasts can be enlarged by using her own fat.

This is where the patient will undergo normal liposuction but rather than throw it away, the surgeon processes the fat and injects it back in small quantities into both breasts. This way a patient could avoid implants and have just their own natural tissue. Unfortunately, not all of this fat will "take" or stay behind so a patient may find she loses up to half of it in the weeks after surgery. This option is more expensive usually as it takes longer in the operating room and has a less predictable outcome than using an implant. In order to significantly upsize a patient, several rounds of fat grafting would be needed, meaning the patient would have to have several expensive surgeries. For this reason, most patients who want a significant breast augmentation will stick to implants.

There are 6 questions a patient must answer before undergoing breast augmentation surgery or a "boob job". The surgeon will often nudge the patient towards the better option if there is one.

1- Size

This is probably the most important question a woman must decide prior to breast augmentation. Unfortunately, implants don't conveniently come in cup sizes. The fact is bra cup sizes vary greatly between manufacturers, so they are a poor way to decide anyway. Instead implants come in "c.c."s or milliliters. To make things more confusing they come in an array of different shapes and heights. Communication with your surgeon is critical – what I think is natural and you think is natural may be two very different things.

What I encourage patients to do is bring photos of what their goals are. We will usually decide on a range and understand that allowing the surgeon to have a little bit of artistic license is always best.

With size there is certainly a sweet spot. There is a certain range of implant that will fit underneath your breast like a glove providing natural results and longevity of those results. If we exceed the size that fits in that pocket, we may over time see some changing in the results as the implant drifts down with gravity – the most common is "bottoming out". Meaning an increase in the distance between the fold and the nipple that looks unnatural.

Some patients will certainly take that risk in order to achieve a full-sized breast, but she should be aware if she is exceeding this sweet spot and increasing her chances of wanting or needing revision surgeries in the future. For many larger transgender women, they can accommodate a large implant so this can be less of an issue.

2- Silicone vs. Saline

Silicone got a bad reputation in the 90s and was taken off the market briefly for concerns that it would cause disease if it ruptured. Happily, it was found that these claims were untrue and its back on the market and by far the most common implant used around the world. The FDA when re-approving it introduced a few stipulations. Patients must be over the age of 22 and they must monitor the implants as it is often impossible to know whether or not the implant has ruptured. Patients are advised to get an MRI at 3 years after they are placed and every 2 years thereafter. It is estimated that in reality very few women actually do screen their implants as MRIs are expensive and often not covered by insurance if the implants were considered "cosmetic".

Silicone has a few advantages over saline- firstly there is less chance of rippling. Rippling is a problem usually thinner girls will have with larger implants whereby the edges of the implant are visible underneath the skin. In addition, silicone may feel softer and more natural. The main advantage saline has is it is cheaper and there is no chance it will be ruptured, and a patient not know about it. When saline implants rupture, they go flat quickly, and a patient will be lob sided.

3- Position of the Incision

There are three main options for placement of the incision. The most common approach is to gain access for the implant via an incision in the fold underneath the breast – the infra-mammary (IMF) fold.

The next most common is an areolar incision and the third is an incision in the axilla or armpit. The trans-umbilical or belly button approach is rarely used. These incisions will usually be small and heal very well. When larger implants are being used and in a girl with small nipples to begin with, usually the IMF will be the safest approach. Preferences vary from surgeon to surgeon.

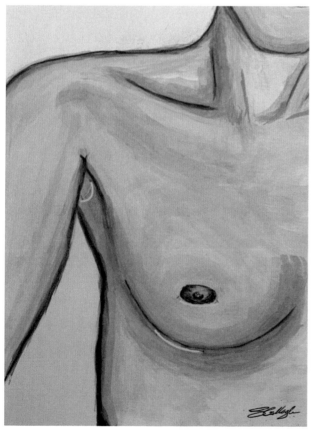

Figure 96 Three possible incision positions, axillary (armpit), Peri-areolar (around the nipple) and Infra-mammary (under the fold).

4- Position of the Implant

Most breast augmentation patients in the United States will have their implants placed either under the muscle or more commonly partially under the muscle. This is mainly because there is a decreased chance of developing a capsular contracture.

Capsular contracture; whenever a foreign body is placed into the body the body walls it off with a capsule- no big deal. The problem is however if that capsule begins to contract or tighten around the implant it causes hardening, displacement and sometimes even pain. The chances of this happening with modern techniques are less than 5% of patients.

Many transgender women in my experience, may benefit however in placing the implant underneath the breast itself and not the muscle. There are a couple of reasons for this. Firstly, as I mentioned cleavage is difficult to create in many transgender women so placing the implant underneath the muscles may make this problem worse as the muscles push the implant away from the middle of the chest. Secondly as mentioned above the breast may have a tuberous appearance meaning the lower part of the breast may not have a rounded-out appearance and we must instead rely on the implant to help create that roundness therefore it is best not hidden underneath the muscle.

5- Surface of the implant

The two options available here are smooth vs. textured implants. Textured implants were thought to decrease the chances of capsular contracture (above). They have however been falling out of favor recently because they have been linked to a new very rare disease. This is breast implant associated anaplastic Large Cell Lymphoma. The good news is this disease is usually adequately treated by removal of the implant and the capsule around it. It appears to be more common with the textured implants so many surgeons therefore are placing smooth implants instead.

6- Shape of the Implant

In the USA there are 2 major choices here the shaped implant or the round implant. The shaped implants were designed to have a more tear drop shape and perhaps avoid the "Baywatch" effect of a rounded shape to the breast. However, with gravity in my opinion round implants will take on a teardrop shape anyway when the patient is upright. I therefore haven't noticed an advantage with these implants. Some disadvantages with a shaped implant are a larger incision is often needed and they can change position and spin upside down in the chest requiring a surgery to correct that.

Breast Lift / Mastopexy

Depending on the shape of the patients breast an additional surgery may be recommended in order to improve the appearance.

A breast lift is generally for patients who have "sagging" or ptosis of the breasts.

Usually it means there is too much skin there which needs to be removed so the nipple can be lifted up to a better position and we can get a rounder, fuller shaped breast.

The only way to get rid of extra skin is to put incisions on the breast itself. These can vary, depending on how much skin we need to remove.

In the case of transitioning patients this surgery is rarely needed. Usually the main complaint is lack of breast tissue development, so sagginess is rarely a complaint. Exceptions may be if the patient has lost a lot of weight and has deflated breasts. Then like any other weight loss patient she may have excess skin she desires to have removed.

There is one other circumstance that a mastopexy might be useful to a transfeminine patient.

Sometimes as new breasts develop, they will have a "tuberous" appearance. What this usually means is that the lower half of the breast will not develop well. They might have a tight high fold the nipple "spills" over and ends up in an unusually low position.

In the majority of patient's breast augmentation alone will be enough for that patient, however in some a breast lift or mastopexy may help improve the appearance. This will usually be done at the same time as the implant placement.

Risks- What can go wrong after Breast Augmentation

Breast Augmentation is a quick procedure that usually results in very happy patients. However, like any surgery there are always risks. Here are the big ones.

Infection- your surgeon will be extremely careful when putting in an implant to make sure there is no infection. This is SO incredibly important with implants. If your body gets an infection without an implant usually antibiotics will work. However, with the implant infected often times that infection won't go away until the implant is removed! This of course can mean another surgery and possibly time with no implant in at all. The chance of this complication is less than 1%.

Hematoma- Hematoma or bleeding can happen in the days and weeks following surgery. For most patients this will mean there is a lot of bruising and asymmetrical swelling usually seen on just one side. Your surgeon will decide with you if the best thing is to wait it out or do another surgery. Rarely the patient may need an emergency surgery to stop the bleeding.

Changes in Sensation- A small percentage of patients will notice a decrease in sensation after placement of an implant. In most this will improve in the months after surgery.

Asymmetry – Often times as already discussed asymmetries that are there before the surgery will be magnified after surgery. While every surgeon will try to match things as well as possible and likely use different sized implants this is unfortunately not an exact science.

Rupture – Every patient getting implants should realize that that particular implant is very rarely for life and we know she is automatically signing up for a surgery later in life for a number of reasons

It is estimated that the risk of rupture is approximately 1% per year. Some surgeons will advocate switching them out at 10 years. In general, I recommend if its not broken don't fix

it. However, statistics show that most patients undergoing breast implants will undergo at least one other breast surgery at some time in her life.

Recovery After surgery

Breast augmentation takes approximately 45-90 minutes to perform is done as an outpatient with most patients returning to work in 1 week and full activities in 6 weeks.

Implants generally take some time to "settle" and may appear to "ride high "initially.

Each surgeon will have their own recommendations on whether massage or special bras are needed but most advise avoiding an underwire bra until incisions are completely healed.

Fact- Breast Implants do not need to be switched out at 10years unless there is a problem.

6. Voice feminization

By Vartan Mardirossian MD FACS

WHAT IS VOICE FEMINIZATION SURGERY?

Voice feminization (aka Wendler glottoplasty or Vocal Fold Shortening and Retrodisplacement of the Anterior Commissure (VFSRAC)) is a procedure that benefits patients who desire a higher pitched, more feminine voice. During a voice feminization surgery, the Surgeon shortens and increases the tension of the vocal cords, which produces a higher-pitched and more feminine voice. VFSRAC is a safe and reliable method, that was first described in Korea in 2017, and performed at our practice in more than 50 patients between 2018 and 2020. It is a further improvement of Wendler's feminization glottoplasty that was described in 1992. With this approach, the outer surface of the vocal folds is removed, and they are then sutured together tightly with a very fine permanent suture material to accomplish tightening and the creation of a feminine geometry to the larynx. VFSRAC is not the simple creation of a laryngeal web: the vocal folds are not only sutured together, but the entire anterior commissure of the vocal folds is moved posteriorly to create more tension and thinning of the vocal folds to increase their fundamental frequency. Voice feminization surgery works best for those who have undergone and are willing to continue to undergo, speech therapy. This procedure is usually performed alone and not in combination with other Facial feminization procedures.

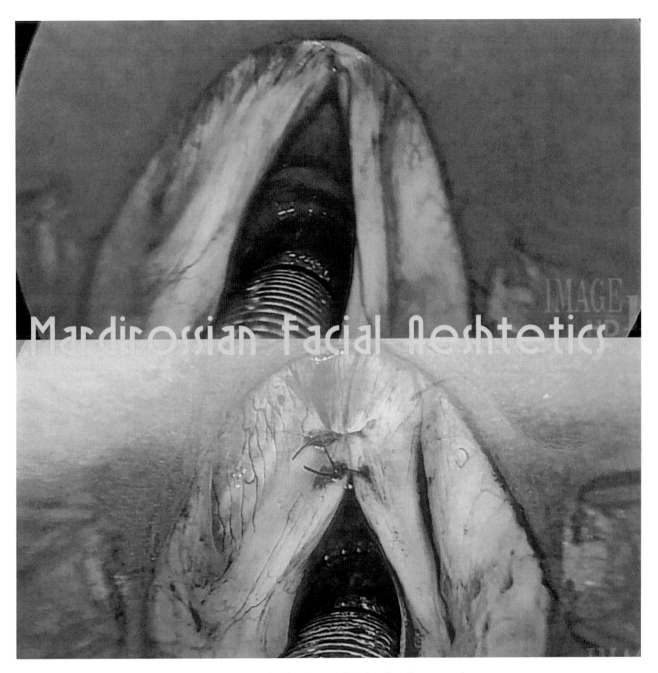

Figure 97 Surgeon's View Immediately after the procedures.

AM I A CANDIDATE FOR VOICE FEMINIZATION?

Voice feminization is about more than simply appearance: it is about how you sound. In fact, part of transitioning involves feminizing the voice. The end result should be a natural, more feminine voice. The surgery itself is minimally invasive, has no skin incisions, and usually involves only the vocal cords. As a general rule, Dr. Mardirossian encourages his patients to start speech therapy prior to the surgery. This way, their baseline fundamental frequency, and speaking pattern can be registered, and the use of postoperative exercises can be reviewed ahead of time.

If you are already working with a speech therapist and would like your voice to have a higher pitch, then you are probably a candidate for voice feminization. However, many times speech therapy alone can improve your ability to produce a higher-pitched voice. The voiced speech of a typical adult male will have a fundamental frequency from 85 to 180 Hz, and that of a typical adult female from 165 to 255 Hz. Women's voices are more melodic while men's voices are more monotonous. In speech training terms, this means that women have an overall higher voice frequency, and they change the frequency of their voice much more frequently than men. Speech therapy teaches the patients to use their voice as a feminine one, regardless of the pitch. The surgery in this sense helps achieve a natural melodic and appropriately feminine-sounding voice.

HOW IS VOICE FEMINIZATION PERFORMED?

The procedure is performed through a narrow 2-cm metal tube that is introduced in the throat through the mouth. The tube allows the Surgeon to visualize and operate on the vocal folds. A microscope is brought into the field, which magnifies the vocal folds and allows for precision work to be performed.

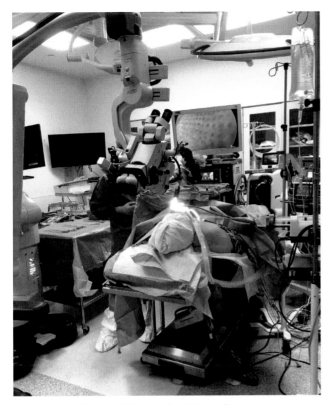

Figure 98 Operating Room Set up

Fig 2: Operating room setup and instrumentation

The anterior third of the vocal folds and the area of the larynx immediately inferior to them is roughened to allow for healing that will retrodisplace the anterior commissure of the vocal folds. In other words, the anterior attachment of the vocal folds is moved posteriorly. To facilitate this, the third anterior of the vocal folds is sutured together with a permanent suture. This process altogether shortens the vibration length of the vocal folds and increases tension, resulting in a higher voice pitch, very similar to how a guitar chord is being tuned.

Bear in mind that the surgical field for this procedure is roughly 5-7 mm in size and at 22-23 cm distance from the surgeon's hands, so it requires exceptional level of attention, surgical micro-coordination and skill. The procedure is performed under general anesthesia and takes about 1.5 to 2 hours to perform.

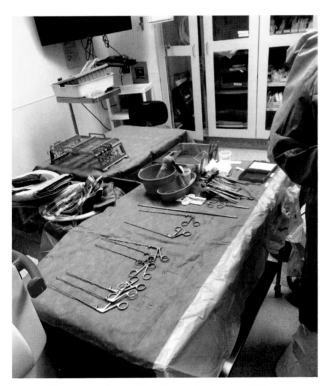

Figure 99 Operating Room Instrumentation

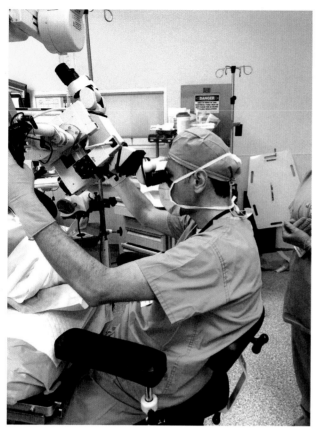

Figure 100 The Procedure requires utmost concentration and skill from the surgeon.

WHY ARE PERMANENT SUTURES USED AS OPPOSED TO ABSORBABLE ONES?

After the procedure, the brain has to get used to the new length and tension at which the vocal folds have to operate. This process of "resetting the system" takes up to six months and is the main source for a hoarse voice after the initial swelling and inflammation of the voice box have resolved.

To understand this process, just think about trying to drive your car by pressing the pedals with your left foot instead of the right one. Not having the fine motor skills, your left foot will be pressing on the pedals way too abruptly to allow a smooth ride. During the process of motor reconditioning of the brain, the permanent sutures allow for a firmer union between the vocal folds and a better chance for success of the operation.

Temporary sutures may absorb prior to the completion of the motor adjustments and therefore compromise the result of the procedure. Permanent sutures will also cause some thinning of the vocal folds in the long run, with an additional increase in voice pitch months and even years after the procedure.

WHAT ARE THE POSSIBLE RISKS FROM THIS PROCEDURE?

Potential complications include bleeding, infection, reaction to the anesthesia, damage to adjacent structures from placement, and use of the surgical equipment: injury to lips, teeth, tongue, larynx, and pharynx. A small portion of patients may experience temporary "numb tongue, altered taste, TMJ syndrome, and dental injury. Potential prolonged or permanent hoarseness, breathing, or swallowing problems are described although rare.

WHAT SHOULD I EXPECT AFTER VOICE FEMINIZATION SURGERY?

Following the procedure, the patient will spend 12-24 hrs under hospital observation, during which the blood oxygen levels will be followed, and the patient's comfortable breathing will be assured before discharge. After voice feminization, patients should remain at complete voice rest for two weeks. Coughing and sneezing should be avoided as much as possible.

After the initial period of complete voice rest, use of the voice can be resumed and increased gradually. Following the surgery, patients often find that their voices are deeper due to the swelling and inflammation of the larynx. It may get worse before it gets better, and it may take up to six months for the roughness to dissipate completely. It generally takes six weeks or so before patients are fully healed and able to reach some of their higher pitches.

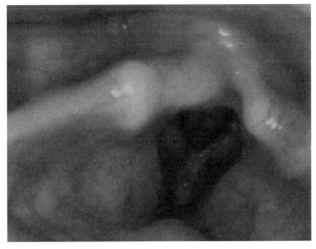

Figure 101 View of the Larynx one month after the procedure.

IS VOICE FEMINIZATION ALONE ENOUGH TO HAVE A NATURAL, FEMININE VOICE?

Keep in mind that most voice feminization surgeries can only truly affect the pitch of the voice, and not the resonance, which can also affect the way a patient's voice sounds. Often times, results are dependent on the success of the surgery along with the patient's effort to undergo voice retraining, much as a singer is taught to use and control higher octaves. Surgeons often plan these procedures based on individual needs, so speaking to Dr. Mardirossian before the procedure is the best way to determine expectations.

HOW LONG WILL MY VOICE FEMINIZATION SURGERY RESULTS LAST?

The results of voice feminization are permanent and cannot be reversed. Since the largest possible portion of the vocal folds has been addressed with voice feminization, no further increase of the voice pitch is surgically possible. As mentioned already, the results from voice feminization surgery are further enhanced with the help of voice training. Please check our website at https://www.palmbeachplastics. com/voice-feminization-surgery-west-palm-beach/ and https://www. palmbeachplastics.com/before-after-voice-feminization-west-palm-beach/ for results and more information about voice feminization surgery.

Section 2

Healthcare for Transmasculine Patients and Non-Binary Assigned Female at Birth Patients

1. Masculinizing Hormones

By Dr Sidhbh Gallagher

Testosterone

For many transmasculine patients, hormonal therapy will be one of the earlier steps in transition.

In the US most patients will be started on injections (testosterone pills are not available). Depending on the type of medication used these are often given on a weekly or every two-week schedule. Patches and gels are also becoming more commonly used, however, some patients may find changes happen more slowly with these transdermal (gels or patches) medications.

Changes with testosterone can happen slowly just like puberty – we are usually talking years not weeks. Raising the dose of testosterone usually won't speed this up but could lead to some dangerous side effects. It is important to discuss specific goals with your hormone prescriber. For example, non-binary identifying patients may not want all the masculinizing effects of testosterone. It is unfortunately almost impossible to pick and choose which effects a patient will get. In these cases, the prescriber will usually start off with a low dose of the hormone. The speed and degree of changes seen vary a lot from patient to patient. Most effects will take 2-5 years to be seen. Often times younger patients may get more effects as compared to patients who started later in life.

What to expect on Testosterone?

Body shape changes

Patients may slowly with time notice that the fat around the hips and buttocks may now be found to form more around the stomach area. Arms and shoulder muscles may increase in size and particularly folks who work out may find that they "bulk up" more easily with time.

Skin changes

Patients may notice their skin become oilier and pores get bigger. Acne can be a problem that is worsened or brought on by testosterone.

Hair

Facial and body hair growth can be a very gradual process. Some patients may also experience thinning of the hair around the temples and male pattern baldness.

Voice

Testosterone can deepen the voice by thickening the vocal chords. As these changes are happening some patients may notice hoarseness or the voice can "break" similar to in puberty. Not all men will get masculinization of the voice and some find speech therapy helpful.

Breasts

The effects of testosterone on breasts size is usually disappointing – some shrinkage may occur but usually not enough to substitute for top surgery. Timing of surgery and testosterone use tends not to be very important as minimal shrinkage usually happens, and the skin of the breasts won't shrink either therefore it usually won't make much difference in the type of surgery needed.

Menstruation

Many patients will notice their periods become lighter and indeed stop completely on testosterone. It is important to remember however that testosterone is not a contraceptive and it is still very possible to get pregnant while taking it.

Sexual changes

Many patients will notice an increase in their sex drive. Also, the sexual experience may change and so too may the patient's sexual orientation. The clitoris will also begin to enlarge. After a while on testosterone some patients may experience "atrophic changes" to the vagina and vulva. These are much like the same changes non-transgender women get when going through menopause. Symptoms from this may include dryness and soreness and sexual difficulties. Other causes need to be ruled out but sometimes estrogen creams can be useful and should have minimal effect otherwise as they are not well absorbed into the body.

Emotional changes

Some trans-masculine patients may notice testosterone can affect their moods and how they relate to other people. Just like any puberty some can find it an emotional roller coaster. It is important to remember mood swings can be normal.

Testosterone and Fertility

Over the long-term testosterone may irreversibly damage the ovary's ability to produce eggs. Transgender men have certainly been able to stop testosterone and get pregnant, but this is not always reliable. Some transgender men will freeze their eggs in order to preserve fertility in the future. Many insurance plans however do not pay for this, it is expensive and there is no guarantee it will work.

Risks of Testosterone

Overall testosterone seems to be very safe when monitored by a physician at the right dose for the patient.

Men have higher risks than women of certain conditions such as high blood pressure and heart attacks. They also have shorter life expectancies so theoretically starting testosterone and taking it long term may bring these issues.

Some patient's blood may become "thicker" (increased red blood cell count) especially in the first few months of taking testosterone. This could lead to increased risk of blood clots, which your doctor will monitor for.

Some patient's cholesterol levels have increased on testosterone also.

It is not exactly known what the long-term risks of cancer are from taking testosterone. Some experts will recommend that the uterus and ovaries be removed within about 5-10 years after starting hormones to decrease any potential negative side effects on these organs.

What checks will I get?

When starting a patient on testosterone a few things need to be taken into consideration. Firstly, what are the patient's goals? Do they have any medical conditions that testosterone may affect? Then once started on testosterone not only the patient's testosterone levels on a blood test need to be taken into consideration but also what progress the patient is making and are there any safety concerns.

Most providers will check labs to monitor the risks outlined above and also testosterone levels at 3 months, 6 months and a year. Once the patient reaches about the midrange for testosterone most providers will monitor it yearly after that. Again, this is however not a one size fits all therapy and patients are usually monitored in the context of what's otherwise happening response and health wise.

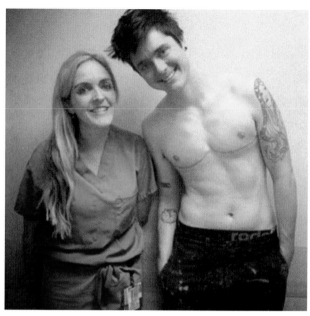

Figure 103 Dr Gallagher and a Masculoplasty patient.

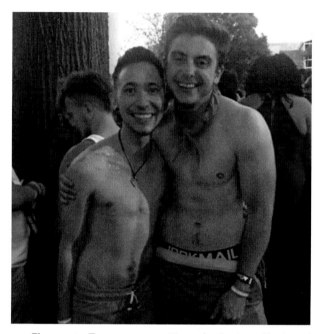

Figure 102 Two awesome Masculoplasty patients enjoying pride.

2. Top Surgery

By Dr. Sidhbh Gallagher

A patient can have top surgery without ever having been on testosterone. Hormones are not right for everybody. For many non-binary identifying patients, hormones are not necessarily part of the transition. However, I am often asked by patients if they should try testosterone for a while, would it possibly shrink things down, and maybe help with the result. The answer to this is dependent on whether you have a small chest or not. If you have a very small chest to begin with, it could possibly make the difference between whether or not you are a candidate for keyhole versus double incision. This is very rare, usually if you have any extra skin at all there, testosterone is going to do absolutely nothing to shrink this down. Indeed, very often testosterone does not really shrink breast tissue much at all. The answer therefore is that it doesn't make that much of a difference, so I don't usually have patients wait.

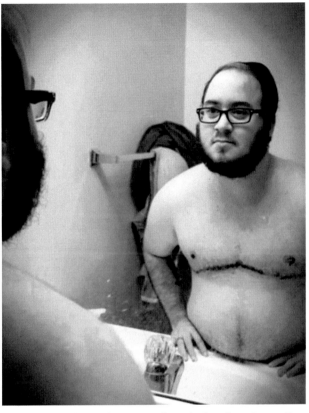

Figure 104 Alexander recovering nicely a few days after Masculoplasty.

Your Health and Chest Binding.

While waiting for this surgery, or if the patient chooses not to undergo it, many people still choose to bind their chests.

Is binding your chest dangerous?

Obviously binding too tightly, and binding during exercise are never good ideas, and are to be strongly discouraged. It is also good practice to give yourself a break from the binder and not wear it 24/7. It's important to get a binder that fits correctly and doesn't pinch or cut into the skin. A common problem, people who bind may come across during the hot months, is the development of rashes underneath the breasts. This is usually due to a fungal infection such as "candida intertrigo". Patients typically will get redness, irritation, and itching which is worsened in hot months when the chest is bound. If you develop symptoms like these your doctor can prescribe either a cream or a powder, however a break from tight binding would usually be recommended. It is very important to note that during exercise your chest needs to be able to expand to breathe properly, and binding should be avoided at this time also.

"Will binding effect the outcomes of my top surgery"

In my opinion as a top surgeon binding doesn't really impact top surgery results negatively. However, in patients who wear a tight garment for a long time, grooving or indentations can appear, typically at the shoulders or underneath the arm just above the breast. These are often permanent; however, they are usually much improved with top surgery.

In rare cases if the breasts are small to begin with binding the chest downwards could potentially turn a candidate for keyhole surgery into somebody who must get a double incision. Patients shouldn't be too concerned about this though, because if there is that much skin there in the first-place, double incision was likely always going to be the best option.

We can therefore conclude that binding in moderation is a safe practice provided the following care strategies are adhered to:

1. The patient needs a break from the binder.

2. It needs to fit correctly and not be too tight.

3. In hot months, be vigilant for rashes that may appear underneath the breasts.

Binding is usually required for just a short time after the surgery between one week and two months depending on the technique used.

Chest options for Assigned Female at Birth Non-Binary Patients

It is critical to remember that a flat "masculinized" chest may not be the goal for everyone. It is very important that patient and surgeon decide what would be most affirming for the individual. As such there are certainly other options. An example of this would be a fairly dramatic reduction in the breast size but not removing as much breast tissue as in a typical masculinizing procedure so that the patient still has some breast mound. The same thing goes for the size and shape of the nipples – we do not have to stick to the typical "male" nipple dimensions. Photos can be really helpful for the patient and surgeon to agree on what exactly the goal is.

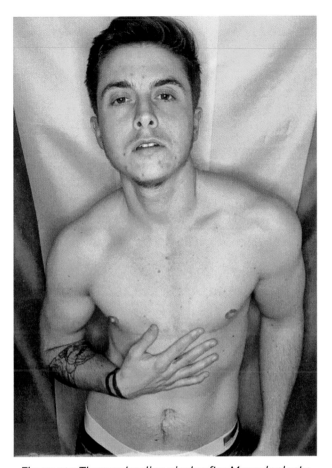

Figure 105 Thomas healing nicely after Masculoplasty.

Top Surgery

Trying to understand the different top surgery techniques and which one will work for you can be very confusing.

The good news is it really just comes down to 2 main techniques a patient must decide between.

1-Around the world the most common procedure is simply removing the breast and the skin on each side- the double incision- and most commonly the nipples come off completely and are grafted into their new position. This procedure goes by many different names including our own name for it Masculoplasty which uses a special internal stitching technique so the patient can avoid drains.

Scars

The vast majority of surgeons will create a horizontal scar, which we try to hide in the fold under the patient's pec muscle to give the most natural appearance. In larger patients or in patients with very closely spaced breasts it may be necessary to continue this scar all the way across the chest to avoid a "central dogear". This is basically a lump that sits in the center of the chest and will never go away or as we call it the "proboscis deformity."

Some surgeons may put the incisions elsewhere such as vertically under the nipple or an anchor-shaped scar or "wise-pattern". The anchor shaped scar was designed for reducing female breasts to lift them and make them "perkier" which of course is not our goal in top surgery. This is therefore rarely used. Sometimes surgeons may put the skin incisions around the nipple, if not much skin is to be removed (peri-areolar) or on

one side (lollipop) or both sides (fish mouth).

With few exceptions the horizontal scar in the fold is the way to go for the most natural results.

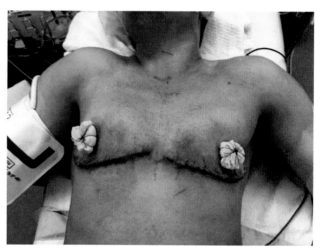
Figure 106 Patient immediately after masculoplasty with typical nipple dressings sewn in place.

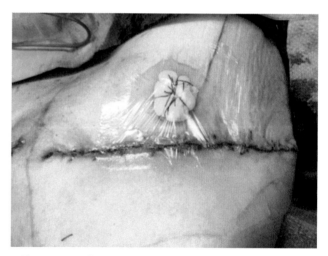
Figure 107 Often the dressing is covered with a plastic layer allowing patients to shower after top surgery.

Nipples

There also can be some differences in how the surgeon deals with the nipple. The majority of surgeons will completely "redesign and masculinize" the nipple. It is removed completely and placed back on as a graft. Some other surgeons may attempt to keep the nipple attached to the body on a "pedicle" or blood supply. Obviously, this pedicle requires that a certain amount of tissue is left behind which can cause unwanted bulk or "moobs." The idea behind doing it this way is to try to preserve more sensation, but this hasn't ever been proven and there is no guarantee it will do that. Therefore, the majority of top surgeons will remove the nipple completely and put it back on as a "free graft".

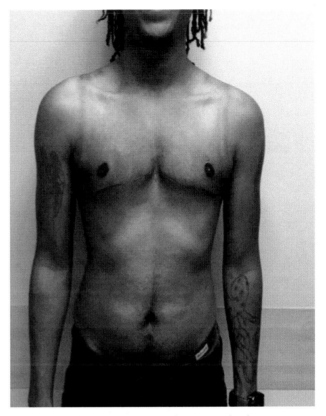

Figure 109 2 months after Masculoplasty

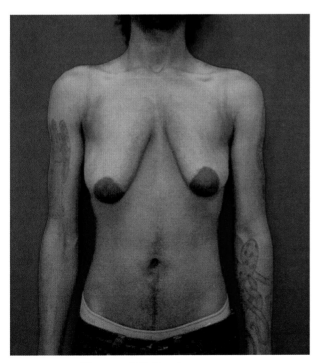

Figure 108 Before top surgery.

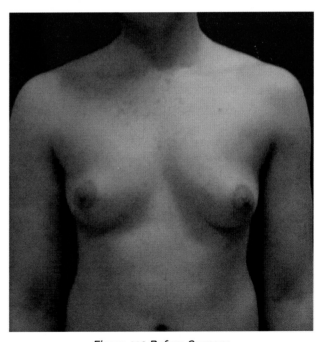

Figure 110 Before Surgery.

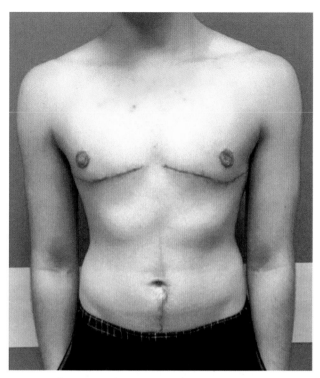

Figure 111 Six weeks after Masculoplasty.

2- Keyhole technique

This is a technique most useful in patients with very small breasts to begin with . A small incision is made disguised in the lower half of the nipple and the breast tissue is removed through this. With this procedure we are hoping that the skin will shrink down over the next few months as no extra skin is removed (the only way to remove extra skin is by placing scars). Often times the surgeon may reduce the size of the nipples as part of this procedure or possibly wait till later to do this. This technique is more likely to require a second procedure for a revision than double incision or Masculoplasty type procedure.

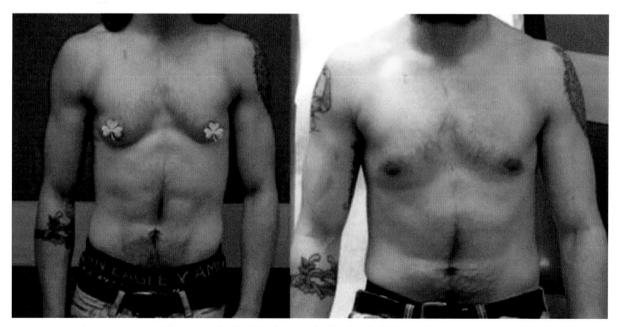

Figure 112 Patient before and after keyhole top surgery.

Keyhole- vs Double Incision- How to Decide.

Is Keyhole even an option for you?

First of all, not many patients are candidates for keyhole surgery at all. Patients have to be pretty small in order to undergo it, this means an A cup or less. This can be very confusing because obviously not many transgender men wear bras! So, what is an A cup? Basically, my rule is you want to have no droopiness in the breast whatsoever. That means the nipple sits above where the fold is. If you have that situation you may be a candidate for keyhole surgery. In keyhole surgery we are making a small incision in the underside of the nipple and through that removing the breast tissue. We are doing nothing to reposition the nipple and hoping that any extra skin will shrink down. How do we know whether the skin will co-operate and shrink down? Unfortunately, we don't know. This depends on your genetics and "quality" of your skin. Much like when a woman has a baby some bellies will shrink down like nothing happened and some will always have loose skin. The younger the patient the more likely they will probably shrink the skin (but this isn't always reliable). About 1 - 2 out of every 10 top surgery patients I see will do very well with either keyhole surgery or a double incision. This often comes down to a matter of personal choice. How important is it to you to avoid that scar?

What if you have both options?

Firstly, you are in a good place – you don't have much tissue to remove so will likely have a great result either way.

One trick I find that is useful in order to help patients predict what their result will look like, is to stand in front of a mirror, and just imagine that we have "sucked all the air" out of your breasts and they are completely deflated, now in your mind's eye, where those nipples are, is exactly where they are going to end up. There is not much we can do in keyhole surgery that will move them. A problem is that often in a "female" chest nipple are more closely spaced and sit a few inches lower than in a "male" chest. If we just deflate everything, sometimes the eye can catch that, and it may look a bit unnatural. Also, often if you need a nipple reduction, that may have to happen at a second surgery.

Keyhole is NOT necessarily the easier option

There can be a misconception that just because we avoid the scarring in keyhole it's an easier recovery. We have found that surprisingly the opposite is often true.

1- Studies have shown that patients are much more likely to want or need revisions after keyhole as opposed to double incision or Masculoplasty.

2- A binder is needed for much longer after keyhole (usually 2 months vs. a week). Fluid collections are a real problem with keyhole as we are not able to put in the special quilting stitches, we use in Masculoplasty and instead must rely on the outside compression to keep the fluid down.

3- It takes longer to see results. With Masculoplasty we are beginning to see a nice flat chest immediately after surgery. With keyhole it can take months especially if the patient develops fluid collections. Waiting for the skin to shrink down requires a lot of patience.

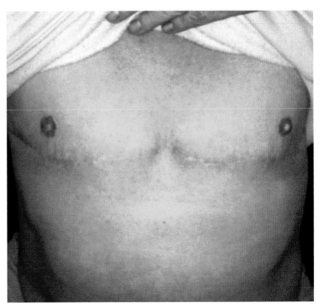

Figure 113 Patient 8 months after Masculoplasty - depending on a patient's genetics the scar often fades to become barely detectable.

Still on the fence?

For some patients this can be an agonizing decision. Most importantly listen to your surgeon- if they are guiding you one way or another – take the hint!

Think bigger picture – your chest is for life. What will your chest look like in 2 years' time? The scars from double incision will be faded whereas with keyhole those nipples may still be too low and closely spaced and actually may look less natural.

If you want to go with keyhole – go for it and accept that you are more likely to want a revision and an enormous amount of patience is required waiting for that skin to shrink down. You can always convert to a double incision procedure later but obviously you can't reverse a double incision to keyhole.

What's the deal with drains?

Drains can cause a lot of confusion. Most surgeons still place them for double incision type top surgery. Are they really needed?

Why are drains placed anyway?

Drains are placed to get rid of fluid (serum) that your body produces whenever a space is made (in this case where the breast tissue has been removed). If that fluid is allowed to collect in there it will cause swelling that can take a long time to go away and may get infected.

What are the downsides of placing drains?

Patients hate drains with many patients complaining that they are the most uncomfortable part of the process.

If drains are placed, they must stay in until they stop draining which is usually about a week (or longer!). It can be annoying having them hanging out of the chest till then and make showering difficult or impossible.

Getting the drains out can be uncomfortable and requires an extra trip to the office.

Drains aren't fool proof – if they accidentally come out too early or fall out the space is still left behind which can lead to seromas anyway.

If drains are left in for a long time, it is thought that bacteria can "crawl" up there and cause infections. For this reason, most surgeons will keep patients on antibiotics while the drains are in. Antibiotics can cause their own problems such as diarrhea and fungal infections.

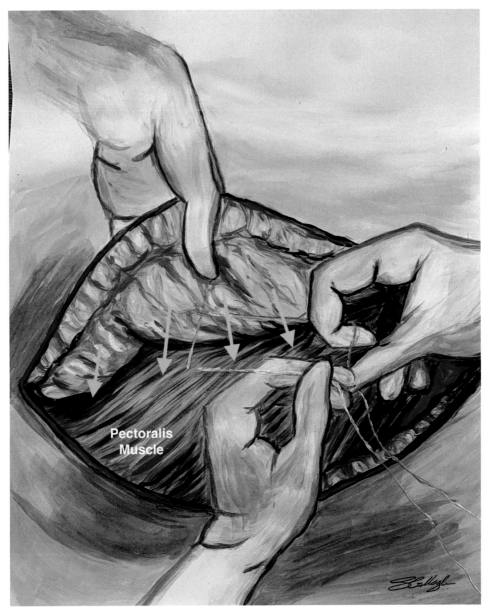

Figure 114 The secret behind the drain free Masculoplasty technique is to place multiple "quilting" stitches on the inside so there is minimal space left for fluid and blood to gather and no need for a drain.

How does Masculoplasty / drainfree surgery work?

If there is no space left behind there is no need to place a drain. To simplify we get rid of the space by using a technique of placing multiple internal stitches to "tack down" the tissue and eradicate dead space.

This technique has been shown to essentially eliminate the risk of significant seromas and also decrease the risk of hematoma.

If your top surgeon however is not comfortable leaving out the drains it is best to listen to them as you want to get the best possible result in their hands.

With Drains

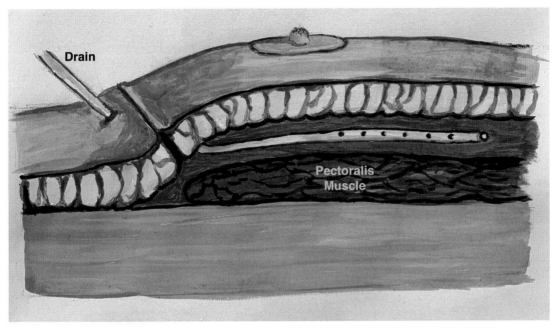

Figure 115 Side view of a patient after mastectomy.
A drain is placed in the space left behind (green) when the breast tissue is removed.

Without Drains

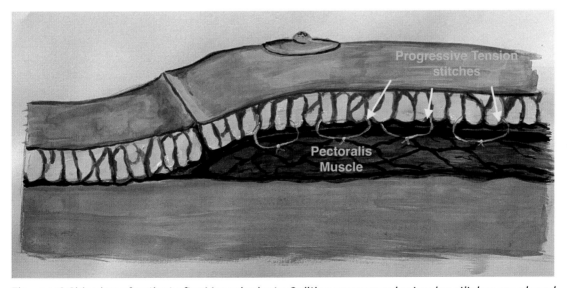

Figure 116 Side view of patient after Masculoplasty. Quilting or progressive tension stitches are placed after mastectomy to eliminate space, so no drain is needed.

Nipples or Not?

Most patients coming for top surgery will know exactly how they feel about having nipples or not. About 15% of my patients have dysphoria surrounding their nipples and the more affirming procedure for them is just to create a nipple free chest.

As long as this is a well thought out choice this is of course very reasonable.

I do like patients to know however that if they DO want nipples in the future they usually look best if made in the OR from the patient's own tissue. I have had some folks wonder if they would be better off just getting tattoos instead of nipple grafts. In those cases, we look through before and after pictures so the patient can decide for themselves. If a patient does however decide to go nipple free – this is a simpler procedure usually lasting 1.5 hrs. instead of 2 hrs. The recovery is also easier as the patient does not have to come back so soon for bolster removal and doesn't have to do nipple care in the first 2 weeks.

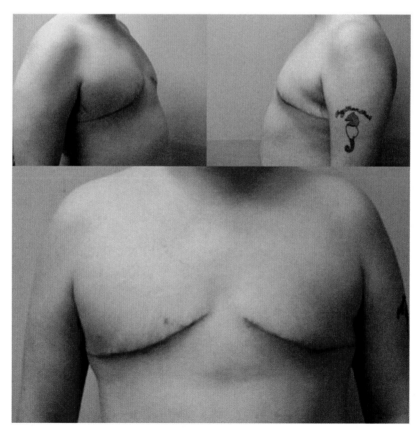

Figure 117 Patient who chose not to have nipples reconstructed.

How to get an idea of what your result will be

One way to figure out how things may turn out is to look through your surgeons before and after pictures. Find somebody who has a before closest to you and this will likely be your result or similar.

If you are planning to go with keyhole, you can get a rough idea of the final result by imagining the breasts were just emptied out and there is a little shrinkage of the skin. The shrinkage varies a lot from person to person.

For Masculoplasty we always try to land the scars in the most natural place possible. For lower BMI patients we can often get these in the fold underneath the pec muscle. In larger folks or patients who have lost a lot of weight this can be trickier. We need to remove the tissue, so we have to have the scars follow where that is. In larger folks this can often be in the shape of an upside-down V across the chest.

Take a look at where the tissue to be removed on the chest is and this will give an idea as to what shape the scars will have.

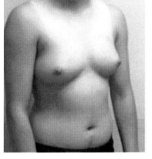
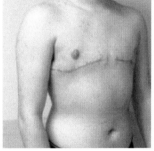
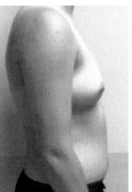
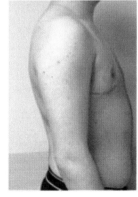

Figure 118 Finding patients who had similar "before" pictures to you will be a good way to predict how you will look after surgery.

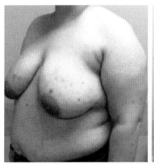
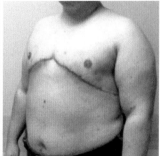
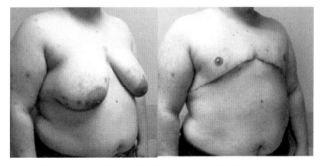

Figure 119 Higher BMI patients will often have downward slanting scars.

In general, I also prefer straighter lines for the chest incisions rather than curved "u-shaped" scars.

If the breasts are spaced close together or in patients with larger BMIs, the scar likely will have to meet in the middle.

If the breast tissue extends a lot to the sides or wraps around the back likely some of this tissue will still remain after surgery. Patients who have chests like this are at higher risk of "dog ears" and are more likely to want a revision surgery later.

What is a dog ear?

A dog ear is tissue that sticks out like a pyramid at the end of a scar. Patients do not like these because they look un-natural and can even poke and rub with clothes. With top surgery it's possible to get them either out at the sides (more common) or in the center or the chest. Some amount of dog ear is very common in the first few weeks and months after surgery as swelling goes down. If the dog-ear doesn't go away by itself an additional surgery is needed to get rid of it usually. The good news is compared to the first surgery it is quick and easy.

Preparing for Top Surgery

Hormones

Thankfully surgeons are now beginning to understand that many folks who need top surgery may never want or need to be on testosterone. Therefore, this is not a WPATH requirement and rarely an insurance requirement.

We do however know that testosterone shrinks breast tissue so patients often ask if they should wait to see what it does for them before proceeding with surgery.

The full effects of testosterone on breasts takes probably a couple of years to kick in and unfortunately patients may find the effects disappointing. Testosterone will do nothing to reduce skin, so patients don't have to wait usually before having top surgery. The only exception may be for a very small chested patient who is on the fence between masculoplasty and double incision. These patients could potentially be swayed one way or the other after testosterone use.

In our practice we typically don't stop testosterone around the time of surgery and believe it's safe to continue as usual.

Screening

It is recommended that patients undergo a screening mammogram after the age of 40 or sometimes earlier depending on family history of breast cancer. Patients may be reluctant to do this as it's often dysphoric and "doc if they are coming off anyway".. Unfortunately, however 1 in 8 women get breast cancer so this is a very important step. If something shows up on the mammogram, we need to know about it before surgery as there are very specific steps, we must first follow to ensure the safest course. All breast tissue removed is usually sent off at the time of surgery to be on the safe side. There currently are no guidelines as to how transgender men should be screened after top surgery. I recommend that patients should follow the recommendations for non-transgender men. Screening mammograms are not needed but any lump found must be investigated. Top surgery will never remove 100% of breast tissue.

Letters

WPATH requires just one mental health professional letter for a patient to undergo top surgery.

Losing weight Before Surgery

Ideally if a patient plans to undergo significant weight loss this should be done before surgery. In this way your surgeon will be able to remove more unwanted skin and probably get you a better result. However smaller amounts of weight such as 10-20lbs won't have much effect really. It is important however that the patient's weight is stable before surgery. Meaning we do not want the patient to be actively trying to lose weight as they will not heal properly. Patients who have lost a significant amount (such as those undergoing bariatric surgery) should wait 6 months after losing weight for this reason.

Considerations for overweight Patients

In an ideal world a patient should not be obese before surgery. This however is not always possible and it's my philosophy that often times the benefits of surgery outweigh the risks. These benefits not only include relieving dysphoria but also the physical problems such as back pain and binding problems. We recently published our Masculoplasty outcomes from my practice where 55% of our patients were obese.

These obese patients didn't have a statistically significant increase in complications (however the super morbidly obese folks did). Therefore, in my practice I like to assess each patient on an individual basis and don't have a strict BMI cut off. Very overweight folks should know they are at slightly increased risk of complications like infection. If a patient is diabetic or has other medical problems its crucial to optimize these before surgery. In addition, "dog ears" are more likely and the chances of needing a revision are also more likely. Often times it is best to make the incision meet in the middle to avoid a lump being left behind in the center of the chest. Overweight patients are also more likely to have sleep apnea which may require an overnight stay in hospital after surgery as these patients can be slower to wake up from anesthesia.

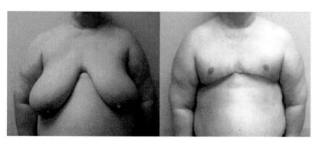

Figure 120 Higher BMI patient before and after Masculoplasty.

Smoking

Smoking anything before top surgery is a no-no.

This is because we are removing the nipples and replanting them, so they are surviving off delicate little blood vessels over the next few weeks. Each time we smoke the blood supply can be "cut-off" so it's one of the surest ways to "kill a nipple". I always remind patients that their chest is for life so making sure they are off cigarettes completely 6 weeks before and at least 6 weeks after surgery is worth it to ensure the best results. It's unclear what vaping does to healing but nicotine is known to be bad for healing (this unfortunately means that even patches are out). Smoking anything increases carbon monoxide in the blood stream, which is also bad.

Diabetics

Diabetics have a tougher time unfortunately healing and we see wound dehiscence (wound opening up) and infections way more commonly in these patients. It is critical to make sure blood sugar levels are as well controlled as possible around the time of surgery to ensure best results. Surgeons will want to see the patient's A1C results which gives an idea of how blood sugar control has been over the proceeding few months this will give an idea of how safe it is to proceed.

Being Otherwise Prepared

Top surgery is such an important step its critical to make sure that now is the time. How is your mental health? Top surgery can be stressful and very anxiety provoking – are you in a good place to proceed? Are you going to be able to do your part to look after nips or should we wait till a better time?

You will need your three "P"s

1. Person- Not only are you going to need somebody for psychological support around surgery, but you will need someone to drive you home, drive you to follow-up appointments, fill your prescriptions reach for that thing of the top shelf…

2. Place-More importantly for folks travelling in but usually a patient can leave about 2 hours after surgery, so you need a safe comfortable place to recover.

3. Pennies – Surgery is expensive business. Even if you have saved up for the price of surgery or

insurance will cover don't forget other unexpected costs may pop-up (deductibles, prescriptions, uber rides, hotels). Also, you won't be working for at least 2 weeks after surgery (6 weeks for strenuous jobs) do you have a plan for this?

What to expect the Day of Surgery

Obviously different surgeons will have different practices but below is a rough guide of what to expect on the big day.

Most patients are asked to show up an hour or so before surgery. Typically, the nursing staff will have you change into a gown and put in an IV line. Next you will meet your anesthesiologist (remember to talk to them about any concerns from previous anesthesia). Your surgeon will typically do some marking on the chest and pretty soon its show-time.

Patients are completely asleep for this surgery and most agree it passes in an instant and before you know it you are sitting in recovery with a compression vest over a nice flat chest. Top surgery usually takes about 2 hours.

In my practice I place lots of numbing medicine while you are asleep as a "block" so usually the pain is not too bad after surgery. Most folks rate it less than a 4 out of 10. Your buddy will pick up prescriptions and once you are able you get dressed and go home. Patients who live a long drive are encouraged to stay nearby for the first 24hrs at least for 2 reasons – the drive can be very rough after anesthesia also if there were any problems after surgery it's good to be close by.

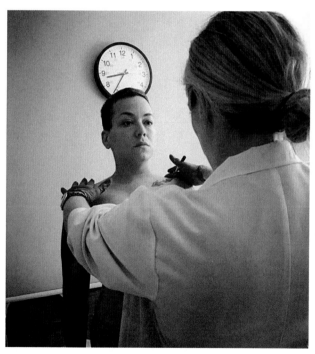

Figure 121 Dr Gallagher marks a patient, Tyne before surgery.

What happens the breasts that are removed?

To be on the safe side, most surgeons will send the breast tissue to the lab in order to ensure there are no surprises like cancerous or pre-cancerous cells.

Recovery from top surgery.

As a general rule I tell patients that they won't feel back to normal for about 6 weeks after top surgery. Even though there are less incisions keyhole requires longer binding and can, even though there are less incisions to heal, feel like a longer recovery. For both surgeries it can take a few months to start seeing the final results as there will be a lot of swelling and nipples in particular can look very strange initially.

In the first few days after surgery patients typically won't want to move their arms round much and will be acting like a "T-rex".

Lifting and Mobility

Patients will be able to move around the house, feed themselves and go to the bathroom but any sort of heavy lifting is out. No more than 10lbs is recommended. Listen to your body it has a great built in warning system, if it hurts, don't do it.

Most patients feel exhausted and "gross" in the first couple of weeks after surgery.

Driving

In order to drive the patient must be completely off narcotic medication and able to make sudden movements. For most folks this is at least a week but more commonly 2.

Sleeping Position

As long as it's comfortable the patient's sleeping position doesn't matter too much. Many patients will prefer sleeping on more pillows than usual or even in a recliner. Sleeping on the back for the first couple of weeks is typical and then slowly side sleeping can be re-introduced. Belly sleepers find this time of recovery toughest. The rule is just sleep whatever way is comfortable.

Work

The soonest folks return to work would be one week after surgery but typically 2 weeks are needed. If heavy lifting or a lot of reaching / strenuous activity is part of the job up to 6 weeks may be needed off work.

Working Out

Gentle walks are a good idea in the first few days after surgery but remember you will get tired quickly. Lower body low impact work outs can usually begin about 2 weeks after surgery and patients are released to regular working out at 6 weeks. Patients who avoid overhead (shoulder) exercises for 6 months after surgery seem to have better appearing scars so if that's an option, I encourage patients to do that.

Compression

Your surgeon will usually provide you with a compression vest in which you will wake up typically.

After Masculoplasty patients require compression for just one week or less after surgery although many surgeons require longer. We prefer patients to wear it 24/7 to decrease swelling however breaks are of course allowed.

Showering

It's up to the patient's surgeon when showering is allowed. Sometimes patients have to wait a week or more (for drains to come out).

In our practice both keyhole and Masculoplasty patients have waterproof dressings underneath the compression vest so whenever they feel strong enough a shower is possible. For most this is 2 days after surgery.

Fact: 6 weeks is the typical down time before strenuous activities can resume.

The Months after Surgery

In the weeks and months after surgery patients will often have larger areas of numbness over the chest. As a general rule these areas of numbness will shrink over the first year so that everything begins to feel normal again. Sensation will come back in the nipples typically also during this time. Some patients will notice weird sensations in the chest during this time such as "lightning bolts" of pain that vanish quickly. We attribute this to the nerves "waking up".

Travelling in for FTM and Non-Binary Top Surgery

Consultations for patients coming in from out of town can usually be done via phone or video conference. This will save the patient the extra trip.

The patient may need a breast exam from their own doctor and possibly a mammogram before travelling in, in order to avoid any surprises that may lead to us cancelling surgery. Patients with other health problems may need additional testing to make sure they are safe enough to undergo surgery. This will be discussed on an individual basis.

Time in Town

Each surgeon will have their own recommendations for how long is required in town.

Keyhole patients may be ready to travel home the day after surgery, but double incision patients should plan to stay a little longer due to the nipple grafts.

The fastest turn around for flying in for our procedure, masculoplasty, is usually 4 days. The patient will arrive in typically the day before surgery and meet with the surgeon.

On the 1st-7th day after surgery the special nipple dressing or "bolster" can be removed most patients leave the area the same day as this.

In masculoplasty we never use drains, so we don't have to wait for those to come out. In some cases, if the patient can find a local doctor with experience to remove the bolsters the patient can leave earlier.

For patients driving in from out of town we recommend getting a hotel in town that night (the drive home can be very rough and if there is going to be bleeding it usually happens in the first 24 hrs.).

Follow-up

Visits after surgery are of course up to the individual surgeon.

Typically, we would see patients at 6 weeks after surgery and then 6 months – however flying is of course not mandatory. We are always happy to video conference/ email or chat with postop patients depending on their needs.

Revisions

About 5% of our Masculoplasty patients will opt to undergo some sort of revision or repeat surgery. This is usually something minor like a "nip tuck" done in the office. Remember many studies have shown that patients undergoing keyhole are more likely to want revisions. Typically, this is not done for at least 6 months after the first surgery. This is because the body will continue to improve on

the appearance for at least a year after surgery. Many times, areas of concern (especially the nipples) will fix themselves as swelling goes down and scars improve.

In general, the more surgery we have to do in the first place the more likely we are to need some sort of "nip-tuck". So, we see when we are taking off a lot in the first place (as with larger chests) the likelihood of a revision goes up. The most common types of revisions are scar revisions or fixing "dog-ears" out on the sides of the chest.

All about Nipples

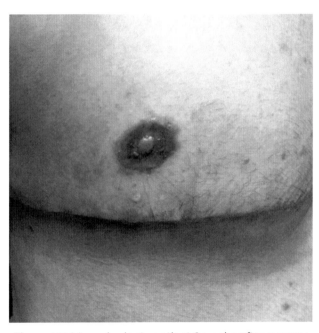

Figure 122 Masculoplasty patient 6 weeks after surgery.

Choosing your nipples

You do have a say in your nipple size and shape after surgery. Many patients will choose to have their surgeon "masculinize" them. What exactly does this mean?

The "male" nipple is different than the female nipple in a few ways"

- The areola is usually oval not round

- The areola is smaller usually around 22mm

- Nipples are spaced wider on the chest

- The nipple has less projection

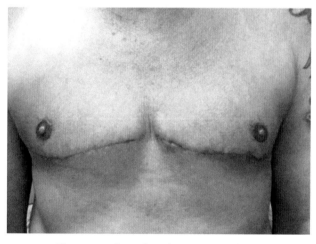

Figure 123 6 weeks after mascuoplasty

Your surgeon will (based on your height and body type) decide during the surgery on the size and shape of the nipples and position them accordingly on the chest.

Masculinization is certainly not for every trans patient and the nipples can be sized and shaped according to what is most affirming for you. Nipple size is one thing you do get a say over!

Some patients prefer not to have nipples reconstructed at all. This option makes your recovery slightly easier and reduces your surgery time itself by about 30 minutes.

What to expect after surgery?

Nipples are the slowest part to heal after top surgery. They require the most care and freak patients out the most!

The First Week

Your nipples are (depending on your surgery) completely removed and grafted or "planted" back on. We sew the dressings onto the chest for the first few days to help everything heal. These are wrapped up then anywhere from 3 days to 9 days (depending on your schedule). These dressings or "bolsters" are removed with the patient awake in the office. This takes 5 minutes and is usually painless. The nipples can look frightening at this point!

They often look purple and flattened. There is often dried up "scabs" around the edges which may "lift up" and look like the whole nipple is falling off. It won't.

Also, blood and other discharge may appear out from around the nipple in the first few weeks. In some patients the entire nipple can even turn black and the top layer of skin "dies off" in a process known as epidermolyis. This can cause a lot of anxiety, but rest assured there is a healthy pink nipple underneath. It is always fine to reach out to your surgeon during this time however if you are worried.

Nipple care

You will be shown how to take care of the nipple until it heals over which is usually about 2-3 weeks after surgery.

Most surgeons recommend a topical antibiotic ointment – such as bacitracin, Neosporin or triple antibiotic. This is often placed on the nipple about twice a day as the nipple will do best in a moist environment. Then gauze or band aids are placed on top to protect the patient's clothes. Typically, the binder isn't needed after the first week but if the patient likes how it feels then they can wear it.

First few months

Nipples heal slowly. In the first few months they usually have a "stuck on" appearance. At about 6 weeks after surgery scar massage of the nipples and other incisions can help.

Patients with darker skin will often have pale or pink patches. These can take up to about 2 years to heal in properly. If after, then the pigment hasn't returned tattooing is a good solution. Interestingly many top surgery patients report a return of sensation after several months. Many of our patients report getting hard nipples in the cold too. In some circumstances the nipples may be overly sensitive in cold weather, but this usually settles down with time.

Scar Care

Unfortunately, the chest is somewhat unforgiving when it comes to scarring. No matter how carefully the surgeon closes the wound some patients will develop raised bright pink scars. Some patients however will get barely detectable fine lines. Much of this is likely due to a patient's genetics. The best predictor of scar healing is how the patient has healed in the past from other incisions.

The good news is with time (up to a few years) the scars will fade and look fine. In fact, scars that have an intense pink color at first often look best in the long run as they will fade to white.

Here are some tips though to help with scarring.

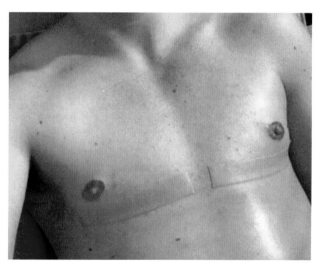

Figure 124 Healing nicely after double incision top surgery (masculoplasty) wearing silicone tape.

Typically, we will want to wait at least 2 weeks weeks before starting scar care to allow the skin to heal. There are many products on the market promising better scar care but unfortunately there is not much science behind any of the products. Rather than wasting money on unproven creams here are my recommendations.

1- Scar massage. This is typically started at around 6 weeks. Using whatever lotion or moisturizing cream the patient usually uses the scar is rubbed in a circular motion with a moderate amount of pressure. This can be done on both the chest incisions and the scars around the nipples. Most patients will do it in the morning when they get out of the shower and maybe at night while watching TV.

2- Limit stretching. There isn't any science behind this recommendation but folks who limit putting their arms over their heads much in the first 6 months seem to have better scars. Typically, this means cutting out overhead work outs.

3- Silicone. The only topical treatment that seems to make a difference to scars (and we don't even understand how, scientifically) is silicone. Both gels and tape seem to work but most patients will opt for the tape as it can be reusable. The more the patient can wear it the better scars seem to do. Your surgeon may be able to supply this, or it is also available online. Some patients may have an allergic reaction to these products so watch out for redness and swelling.

Risks of Top Surgery

Hematoma (bleeding on the inside after surgery)

This would be the most common serious risk after top surgery.

During your surgery the surgeon obviously stops all bleeding however it is possible that the patients may get some bleeding that stirs up after surgery. The most common time for this to happen would be in the recovery room. If the bleeding is significant enough the surgeon will usually take patients back to the operating room to stop it and clear out any blood clots that have formed. If the hematoma is small, it will usually just cause swelling and bruising that will go away over the next few weeks.

Seroma or Fluid Collections

Whenever we remove tissue in the body, it fills the space left behind with fluid. This fluid can be problematic as it causes swelling, can get infected and cause an abscess or it can try to drain out the incisions. This is the reason that drains are left in, in order to remove this fluid. With

Masculoplasty we close down this space so a seroma cannot form. This technique essentially eliminates the risk of large seromas.

Smaller fluid collections may form but they usually disappear on their own in a few weeks.

With keyhole surgery we unfortunately can't close down this dead space with stitches so oftentimes some fluid will accumulate. This can usually be easily and painlessly removed in the office with a needle.

Infections

Some patients may develop redness, pain and swelling round the incision in the first few weeks after surgery. This is only usually seen in overweight patients or diabetic patients. It typically resolves quickly with a course of antibiotics.

Wound Dehiscence

This means opening of the wound. Sometimes a small area of the wound may open up in the first few weeks after surgery. There are usually a few reasons for this -here are the most common.

1-If the patient has not been eating properly after surgery. Especially if they have not been getting enough protein.

2-Smoking

3-Diabetics with poor blood sugar control.

Once the wound opens up the surgeon will typically debride (clean up) any dead tissue and show the patient how to do wound care. This is usually painless. We do not try to close the wound as it will open right up again and possibly get infected.

Depending on the wound size and how well we can control the risk factors listed above it will heal over in a few weeks.

Nipple Loss

Complete loss of a nipple is almost unheard of. As scary as nipples look in the first few weeks, they usually do fine, so we encourage folks to wait. We do sometimes see however that one side may lose some projection as compared to the other.

Oftentimes this is an easy fix in the office to better match them.

3. Bottom Surgery

Authors: Genital Gender Affirming Team - OHSU Transgender Health Program

Chapter Contributors: Carley Putnam, PA-C, Dorian Scull, PA-C, Maureen Steckler, Daniel Dugi, MD, Geolani Dy, MD, Jens Urs Berli, MD
Illustrations by Dr Sidhbh Gallagher

Trans-masculine Bottom Surgery

Gender affirming genital surgery (aka bottom surgery) for trans-masculine individuals includes different options with varying degree of surgical risk and functionality.

Ideally folks can choose the option that best aligns with their gender identity, fulfills their desire for a masculine appearance, and functions in a way that is important to them. A patient's anatomy may or may not allow for all surgical options, and some limitations may exist in the case of other medical conditions. With many different options available, and with many surgeons offering different ways of achieving those options, it can be really overwhelming to figure out what is best for you. Your surgeon can help you sort through the pros and cons of each surgery and assist you in making the right decision. Since your time with the surgeon is often limited, we hope that this chapter can serve as a good preparation for your consultation. Also, if you read this and are a care giver, partner, friend, or family member of someone that is seeking bottom surgery this hopefully will allow you to get a good overview of what bottom surgery means and what decisions your loved one is facing.

Disclaimer: This chapter is written by surgeons and physician assistants at Oregon Health & Science University (OHSU), we have done our best to give you an overview of all the various options that are available, but differences in approach and philosophy between centers and surgeons are common. It is entirely up to you and your surgeon to determine which components and route is best for you.

The chapter is organized in four parts – "Getting ready for surgery and timing", "Metoidioplasty","Phalloplasty" and "Risks & Complications". First, let's look at some common terms used by healthcare providers. Please know that in this chapter we will refer to the anatomy by its anatomical name so that there is no confusion between readers.

Medical Terms

The following list includes terms used throughout this chapter. Please use this as reference as you read through it. It will also be helpful to be familiar with those terms prior to your consultation for bottom surgery.

Burying of clitoris (clitoroplasty)	The procedure in which the clitoris is tucked between the base of the phallus and the scrotum, close to the pubic bone. The clitoris is covered so one cannot see it.
Catheter	A thin tube. Catheters go into your bladder to drain urine.
Donor site	Location on the body where tissue is taken from during surgery.
Erectile device	Device implanted inside the phallus to create an erection. The choices are a semi-malleable device or an inflatable device.
Extrusion	A complication of the erectile device. The implant pushes uncomfortably against the tissues inside the phallus and creates an internal pressure sore. This is most common when staying in a single position for too long, like during air travel.
Flap	Tissue that is moved from one area (donor site) of the body to another site (recipient site). A flap has its own blood supply (blood vessels). It includes skin, fat, fascia, blood supply, and nerves.
Girth	The thickness/circumference of the phallus. Girth can change over time as you heal, or gain/lose fat.
Glansplasty	Surgery to make the glans (head) of the phallus. It gives the phallus the appearance of a circumcised penis with a coronal ridge. This is done using a skin graft from the belly.

Graft	Tissue moved from one area of the body to another. A graft does not have its own blood supply (in contrast to "flap"). A graft receives blood supply from the wound bed (open surface of a wound) it is placed on. Example: skin graft or buccal graft (from inside mouth)
Hysterectomy	Surgical removal of the uterus.
Native urethra	The urethra that one is born with.
Oophorectomy	Removal of one or both ovaries. Some people may choose to keep one ovary for future fertility. Also, a retained ovary is protective if one has future access issues to hormones.
Outpatient	Refers to when one goes home the same day after a hospital or clinic visit/procedure/surgery.
Penile urethra or Shaft urethra	The urethra in the phallus
Perineal masculinization	Surgery to make the genitals appear more masculine. This can include the creation of a perineal urethra, scrotoplasty, burying of clitoris, and vaginectomy.
Perineal urethra (a.k.a. urethral lengthening)	The tube that connects the native urethra to the penile urethra. It is made out of tissue from the inner labia.
Phalloplasty	Surgery to make a phallus using tissue from a donor site.
Revision surgery	Surgery to fix problems or complications.
Scrotoplasty	Surgery to make a scrotum using the skin of the outer labia.
Suprapubic catheter	A tube that comes out the bladder and through the lower belly. It lets one empty their bladder without using their urethra.
Testicular implants	Saline-filled or silicone materials that are the size and shape of testicles. They are put into the scrotum.
Urethra	The tube that urine travels through as it exits the bladder
Urethrogram	X-ray of the urethra

Vaginectomy (a.k.a. colpectomy)	Surgery to remove the vaginal lining to close the vagina. Some surgeons burn the lining to close it.
Void	Urinating

Phalloplasty Timing

The World Profession Association for Transgender Health (WPATH) has set standards of care to determine when it is most safe for a patient to undergo phalloplasty. Keeping in mind that those are guidelines and individual care may vary and is up to you, the surgeon, your mental health professional and often also the insurance company. Usually it is required that you have been on at least 1 year of testosterone hormone therapy and have obtained letters of support from two different mental health providers. Check with your surgeon and your insurance company if a letter from your hormone provider can substitute the second letter. Further if your transition does not include hormones or you have other reasons not to be on them, then the requirement for being on hormones for a year does not apply.

Bottom surgery is by no means a "walk in the park". It is a surgery that often requires a prolonged hospital stay followed by at least one month of careful surgical site care, frequent follow up appointments with your surgeon, and possibly physical therapy to regain strength. Patients also require round-the-clock caregiver needs (often up to one month postop). Therefore, when determining the best time for bottom surgery, one needs to consider their overall health and how well it is optimized, career/job status, family commitments, and ability of friends and family to care for you.

Approaching this step in your transition may seem daunting, however there are patients who successfully prepare and undergo this surgery all around the world. It is ideal to have a multi-disciplinary team at your side that should involve the plastic surgery and urology team, gynecologist, and mental health provider. If there is a need, these providers can interact with your primary care provider and your own mental health professional. Having this professional team and your own caregivers all work together is the best set up for a successful and safe metoidioplasty or phalloplasty. Folks in the community who have already undergone these surgeries are an additional great resource to help you prepare as well but be mindful that every surgeon may have a different care pathway and experiences may vary widely. If possible, try to connect with other patients that had surgery with the same surgeon as you. Also, each person responds differently to the stress of surgery and you can't expect to have the exact same experience as those before you.

Getting ready for surgery

There are many physical health factors that need to be considered when preparing for the phalloplasty or metoidioplasty. Your surgeon as well as your primary care doctor and other specialists can help optimize your preparedness.

Weight: Performing a phalloplasty requires microsurgery to connect small blood vessels and nerves. In cases of excess fat around the waistline the surgery becomes increasingly difficult, and with significant obesity impossible. A BMI is a ratio of height to weight and does not indicate where the fat is on the body. As a rule of thumb: a BMI of 35 and above is too high and weight loss will likely be needed to pursue surgery. However, this decision will be up to you and your surgeon depending on the exam at your consultation. If you do loose a significant amount of weight and have excess skin, then sometimes this needs to be removed at a first surgery. If the amount of excess skin is abundant then it may even limit your options and a shaft-only phalloplasty may be the best route to go.

For a metoidioplasty too much fat at the waistline and the area of the mons can lead to postoperative disappointment as the neo-phallus may not be visible from your viewpoint, and standing urination often is not possible.

Chronic Medical Conditions: Such as high blood pressure and diabetes need to be well-controlled. Your primary care doctor and other specialists can help with this. For patients with diabetes, you must have an HbgA1c of 7 or below.

Tobacco: Use must be discontinued at least 4 weeks prior to surgery (preferably more). Tobacco use *greatly* increases one's chance that they will experience compromised blood flow which can lead to tissue death and loss of the phallus. Other risks include increased chance of postoperative blood clots, pneumonia, and wound healing issue. From a mental health standpoint, we recommend that you stop nicotine products at least 3 months prior to surgery to not add additional stress to an already stressful time in your life. Other recreational substances such as cocaine, methamphetamine, and others can also lead to marked increase in operative risk and should be stopped both before and after surgery.

Mental health: The postoperative period can be very challenging. It is a surgery that requires a long hospital stay, followed by several weeks of limited mobility. You will rely heavily on a caretaker for wound care, cooking, bathing, shopping, errands, and getting you to and from appointments. It is best to prepare coping skills and expectations with your mental health provider and establish a means of communicating in the postoperative period. It is completely normal to have a feeling of regret or depression in the immediate postoperative period, please talk about these emotions and do not feel ashamed of them. They are normal and do not mean that you will feel the same emotions in the long run.

Hair removal: For metoidioplasty there is typically no need for hair removal. If you plan on a phalloplasty and want to stand to urinate, you will need preoperative hair removal in the region of the flap that is used to construct the urethra inside the phallus. This is so hair does not grow in your new urethra which may lead to obstruction, stone formation, and possible need for further surgery. Hair removal on the shaft itself can be done after surgery, so postoperative hair removal for shaft-only phalloplasty or on the external phallus for a patient who wants to stand to urinate is possible. Hair removal options include laser hair removal and electrolysis. Electrolysis takes longer and can be painful but works better for fair and thin hair. Laser requires fewer sessions but is most effective only in patients with dark hair. Hair removal can take several months to a year. This is an important point to consider when planning out the timing of your surgery. At your consult, your surgeon can estimate a hair removal timeline, but the most accurate duration of treatment will come from your hair removal specialist. Your surgeon can show you where hair removal is required at your consult appointment.

Metoidioplasty

The word "Metoidioplasty" comes from the combination of the Greek word *Meta*, meaning toward, *Oidion*, meaning male-gentilia, and *Plastos*, meaning shaping or molding. Initially, as a fetus develops before birth, all the genital parts are the same. Through the influence of hormones, the genitalia then develop differently. With metoidioplasty, we try to use the tissue that *would have* been masculine and rearrange them to create a small phallus.

The first metoidioplasty was performed in the 1970's, roughly 30 years after the first gender-affirming phalloplasty. It was developed as an alternative to phalloplasty - with fewer complications and less time spent in the operating room and recovering.

Metoidioplasty can help folks achieve more masculine appearing genitals, the ability to stand to pee, and maintenance of full erogenous sensation with 1 or 2 surgeries. The main drawback is that the phallus, while natural in appearance, is much smaller than that of a cis-male. For this reason, it cannot reliably be used for penetrative intercourse and will not produce a visible "bulge" in clothing. Under the influence of testosterone, the clitoris enlarges. The primary goal of metoidioplasty is to release the enlarged clitoris from its attachments and make it more visible. Additional goals may include urinating from the tip, creation of a scrotum, removal of the vagina.

Not every person has the same goals of surgery, and a surgery decision will be based on what is important to you and what the anatomy allows. Unfortunately, some patients may not even be a candidate for even a simple metoidioplasty. These patients often have some combination of not enough clitoral growth in response to testosterone, a high BMI, and not enough inner labial skin to cover the phallus. Having to tell a hopeful patient that they likely will not be able to stand to pee, or worse yet – that they are not a good candidate for surgery - is a difficult discussion for both surgeon and patient.

The questions you need to answer are the following:

Do I want to:

· Urinate from the tip of the metoidioplasty?

· Have a scrotum with/without testicular implants?

· Retain the vagina for sexual pleasure?

· Have the ability to give birth?

Sitting to pee can be a very dysphoric experience for many trans-masculine individuals. In addition, it can make folks feel unsafe using the restroom for fear of being "outed" as transgender.

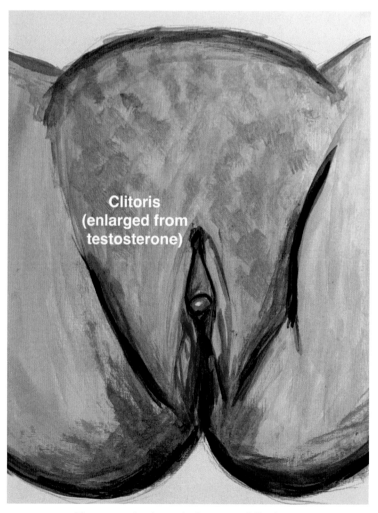

Figure 125 Anatomy before metoidioplasty.

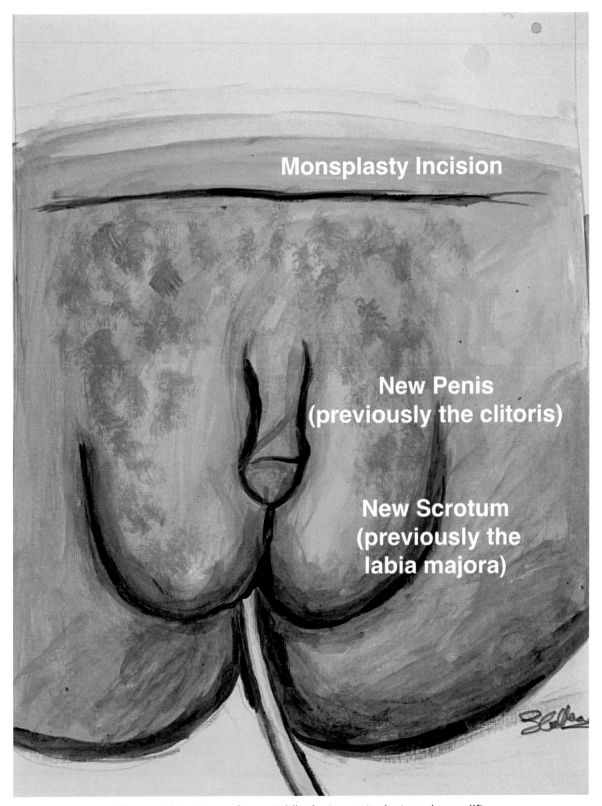

Monsplasty Incision

New Penis (previously the clitoris)

New Scrotum (previously the labia majora)

Figure 126 Anatomy after metoidioplasty, scrotoplasty and mons lift.

For this reason, standing to pee is often one of the main goals of masculinizing bottom surgery. It is important to note though that not all cis-gender males are standing to urinate and that sitting to urinate alone is not gender specific.

In order to achieve standing urination, the urethra needs to be lengthened and redirected through the metoidioplasty. This is called urethral lengthening and is done using your inner labia (labia minora). Some surgeons additionally use *graft* from tissue of the inner cheek to help lengthen the urethra. Luckily, the inside of the mouth heals relatively quickly and without complication (consider how quickly you heal if you by accident bite your cheeks while eating).

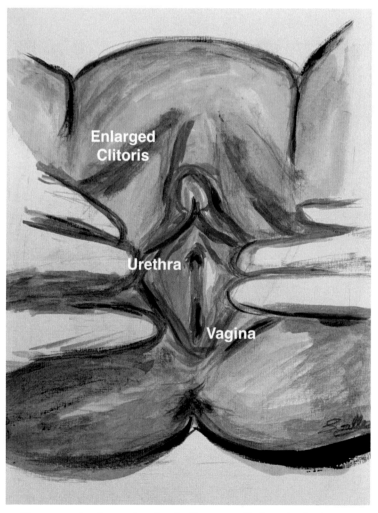

Figure 127 Anatomy showing bottom growth from testosterone.

Unfortunately, with metoidioplasty, not everyone's anatomy will allow for urethral lengthening. An ideal candidate for metoidioplasty with urethral lengthening is someone who has: 1) had good growth of the clitoris from testosterone, 2) has ample inner labial skin (to cover the neo-phallus and lengthen the urethra), and 3) has a relatively low BMI. As a general rule, if you can see the clitoris in the standing position, then you are likely to be a good candidate for urethral lengthening. There is a significant risk for developing a fistula between the urethra and the vagina when lengthening the urethra and this is extremely difficult to repair. For this reason, most surgeons will not perform urethral lengthening without also removing the vaginal canal. But even with that step patients can develop fistulas that are higher up on the metoidioplasty. It should be noted that for patients having a vaginectomy, a prior hysterectomy is also required. Some patients prioritize keeping the vaginal canal for sexual stimulation, childbearing capacity or other reason. For these folks, we recommend *simple metoidioplasty (see below).* This type of metoidioplasty will not allow for standing to pee but has a quicker recovery with less associated risks.

Metoidioplasty Surgery Options:

Based on all the above you can see that there are a few choices you have and hopefully the presented information can help you understand these options better.

Simple Metoidioplasty:

- This involves releasing the clitoris from its attachments and bringing it into a more masculine, forward position.

- It does **not** involve lengthening the urethra so standing to pee will not be possible.

- It does **not** *require* vaginectomy, but this can be done if desired.

- It does **not** *require* hysterectomy if you do not opt for vaginectomy (hysterectomy is required for any surgery involving vaginectomy)

- Most patients can go home on the day of the surgery.

- You will not have to have a bladder catheter

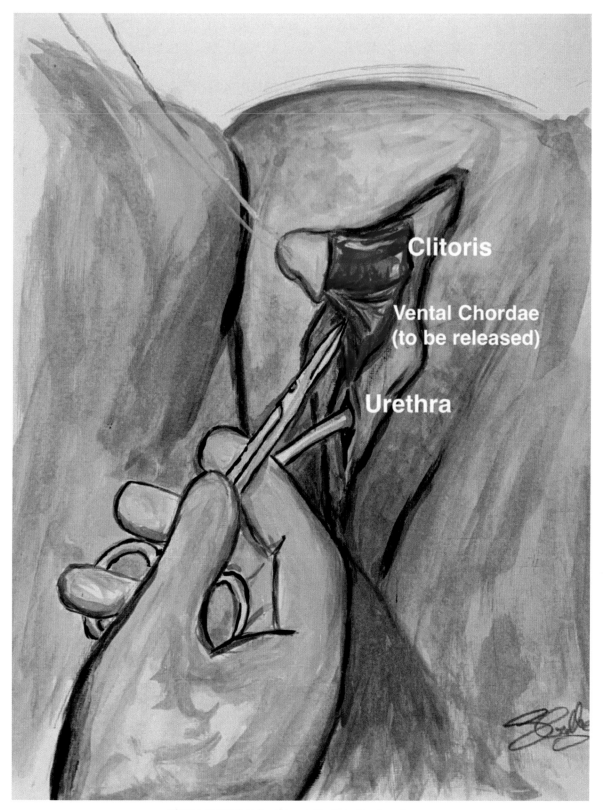

Figure 128 What is released in the simple release.

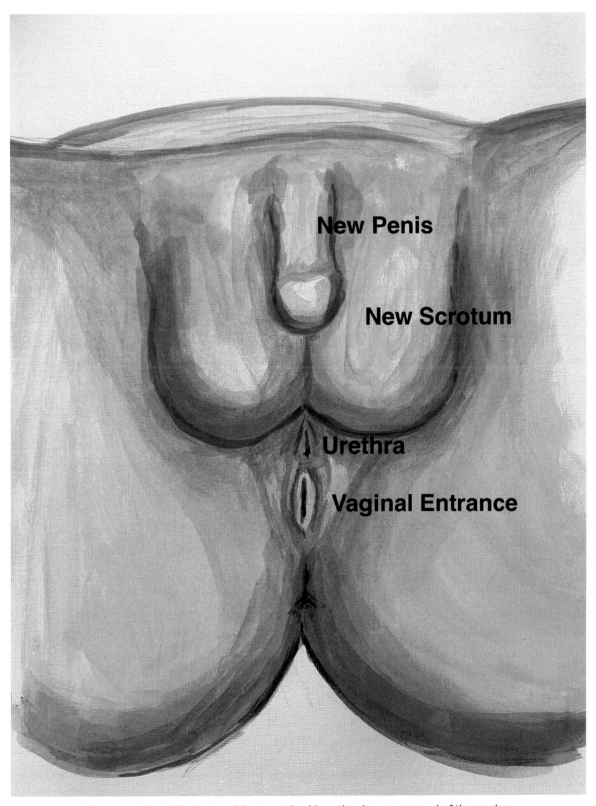

Figure 129 Metoidioplasty without urethral lengthening or removal of the vagina.

Metoidioplasty with urethral lengthening:

- This involves releasing the clitoris from its attachments and bringing it into a more masculine, forward position.

- It also involves lengthening the urethra - with the goal of standing to pee.

- May require a graft from inside the cheeks (buccal graft)

- Lengthening the urethra is associated with higher complication rates and surgical risks

- To reduce risks and surgical complications – vaginectomy and hysterectomy are required by most but not all surgeons.

- To ensure safe recovery after vaginectomy, overnight hospitalization (up to 3 nights) is standard.

- A suprapubic catheter (SP tube) is used to drain your urine while the new urethra is healing

Vaginectomy

This involves removal or burning of the lining of the vagina (colpectomy) and sewing the vaginal canal closed from the inside to the outside (colpocleisis).

- At most centers this is mandatory for surgeries involving urethral lengthening.

- This is because of the risk of an unwanted connection between the urethra and vagina (referred to as a fistula)

- Since the lining of the vagina makes secretions, any remaining vaginal tissue that secretes fluid may cause a mucocele which requires an additional surgery to fix.

Monsplasty

The mons is the natural fat pad over the pubic bone. If it is large, removal may lead to a more masculine, forward, and visible position.

- If this is done, you will have a scar where the skin was removed

- Usually done at the time of metoidioplasty but it can be done later, if needed.

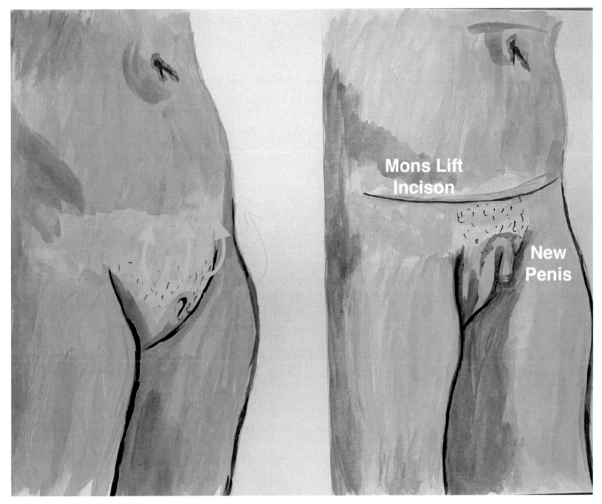

Figure 130 Before and after mons lift

Scrotoplasty

The outer labia are the same tissue as that which develops into the scrotum in cis-gender males. This makes the outer labia an ideal tissue to use to construct a small scrotum at the time of metoidioplasty.

- This is optional and will help to give the genitals a more masculine appearance.

- Testicular implants are saline-filled or silicone-composed implants that can be placed in spaces that we create in each side of the scrotum no less than 3 months after the first surgery, if you wish.

Optional "2nd stage" surgeries

The optional 2nd-stage surgeries are generally cosmetic in nature – helping to create a more masculine appearing genitalia. These surgeries cannot be performed at the time of the original surgery due to risk of compromising the blood supply to the tissues.

Here are some optional 2nd stage surgeries:

VY- advancement:

This 2nd stage surgery involves removing some of the excess anterior outer labial skin to make the phallus stand-out more and create a more masculinized appearance. This requires additional incisions and thus additional vertical scars on both sides of the phallus that range in size from 3-5"

Testicular implants:

This 2nd stage surgery involves placing saline-filled or silicone-filled testicular implants into the scrotum. Many patients, especially physically active patients, find scrotal implants to be bothersome and sometimes have them removed at a later date. Another common complication is that one testicle often "rides high". Sometimes that can be corrected with a revision surgery.

These 2nd-stage surgeries can be done as early as 3 months after the original surgery and can be performed individually or together.

Special preoperative considerations for Metoidioplasty

In addition to the surgery requirements and preparations discussed earlier in this section, here are some special considerations in preparing for metoidioplasty surgery:

Clitoral Pumping

Clitoral pumping (commonly referred to as FTM pumping) is a method to enlarge the clitoris beyond the growth that patients receive from testosterone therapy. This is achieved by placing a vacuum pressurized cylinder over the clitoris and pumping to create suction and increase blood flow to the genitals. If done regularly (many folks say twice daily), it is thought that the tissue around the clitoris will expand and some permanent growth is possible. Patients sometimes ask about how useful clitoral pumping is at increasing clitoral growth prior to metoidioplasty. The answer is – we don't know, and many surgeons advise against it. If the vacuum pressure is too great, it can cause blood vessels to burst, skin to blister, bruising, and damage to erectile tissue.

DHT gel

DHT (Dihydrotestosterone) is a very potent androgen similar to testosterone. Unlike testosterone, DHT cannot be converted to estrogen, thus it has more powerful masculinizing effects. Prior research on treatment of cisgender males with micropenis found that applying topical DHT was effective at increasing penis size. Since the clitoris and the penis are biologically similar, it makes sense that it would also work to enlarge the clitoris, but more studies need to be performed to prove this.

In addition, one of the main side effects of DHT is male-pattern hair loss. We don't know if topical use of DHT would increase hair loss, but we also don't know that it wouldn't. Finally, we have been told that finding DHT gel in the United States has become increasingly difficult and many folks are having to get it from overseas without FDA regulation.

Recovering from Metoidioplasty

The recovery process from Metoidioplasty is largely dependent on how complex the surgery was. Did it involve urethral lengthening with vaginectomy? Was there a monsplasty? The recovery process is also dependent on each individual patient and how well they heal after surgery. With all metoidioplasty surgeries - there will be significant swelling of the phallus initially. This can be quite shocking for many patients. The swelling slowly resolves over the coming months. Typically, by 3 months post-op, most of the swelling has resolved but comes and goes with activity. By 6 months, the swelling should be fully resolved, and the patient will know what their new phallus will look like long-term.

For patients who have had vaginectomy and/or scrotoplasty it is advised to avoid leg spreading and for all patients undergoing bottom surgery it is generally a good recommendation to avoid excess walking in the healing period.

What if a patient decides they want phalloplasty later?

Having a phalloplasty after metoidioplasty is possible. In fact, some surgeons actually use metoidioplasty as a "1st stage" for phalloplasty. However, there are technical differences and if a phalloplasty is the ultimate goal then it is best to have a surgeon who performs the metoidioplasty with this next step in mind.

Phalloplasty

The first phalloplasty was performed in 1936 for a cis-male patient who lost his natal penis. Ten years later, the first gender affirming phalloplasty was performed on a transgender physician by one of his colleagues. Since then, surgical techniques have continued to evolve and improve, but it is still a very complex surgery with a number of risks and complications.

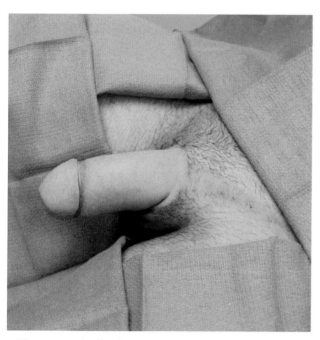

Figure 131 Phalloplasty from radial forearm free flap.

Phalloplasty options

Phalloplasty is not "one" procedure. It includes many different surgical steps that all together make up a "phalloplasty". Those categories are:

- Shaft

- Erectile implant
- Shaft urethra (pars pendula)
- Perineal urethra (AKA pars fixa, urethral lengthening)
- Glans
- Scrotum
- Testicular implants
- Vaginectomy
- Hysterectomy

It is so important that you establish a clear goal for your phalloplasty before undergoing a surgery and to weigh all the risks against the benefits. This also involves considering your fertility desires and your sexual preferences. For example, while for some vaginal intercourse is unthinkable it may be an important sexual function even if that area does not align with their gender identity. In the old days surgeons and mental health professionals questioned patients gender identity when such desire was voiced. However, we do understand today that this was wrong and that your voice is the most important guide in choosing the correct surgery route. A surgical consultation is very stressful, but it is so important that you speak up for yourself. If a surgeon does not listen, then that person is probably not the right surgeon for you. But it is also important to know that some desires that a patient may have are not offered due to increased surgical risk. For example, lengthening the urethra without closing the vaginal canal is not only very challenging but also comes with marked increased risk.

One of the biggest decisions to consider as a phalloplasty patient is whether or not standing to urinate is important to you. If you choose to have the option for standing urination and if your surgeon believes you are a candidate for this, your phallus will be constructed with a neourethra or "new urethra" inside of it. This will be connected to your native urethra (the urethra one is born with) such that it is one continuous outflow tract. At most institutions, if one desires standing urination and a neourethra they must also undergo a vaginectomy to reduce chances of complications. If a vaginectomy is performed, then a hysterectomy (removal of the uterus) is needed as the secretions of the uterus would otherwise not leave your body. When performing a hysterectomy your ovaries are frequently removed as well and with them your ability to have your own

children. Some centers offer you to keep at least one ovary which allows for "backup hormones" to protect your bones and cardiovascular well-being if there is ever a chance that access to testosterone is compromised in the future.

If you decide to have a "shaft-only" phalloplasty then you can choose between three distinct options:

A. Leave genital region untouched

B. Perform a hysterectomy and vaginectomy and scrotoplasty. The native urethra will remain at its location but be visible underneath the scrotum.

C. Retain the vaginal canal but perform a scrotoplasty and burial of the clitoral tissue (Vaginal preservation vulvo-scrotoplasty).

What is a Flap and where does it come from?

The phallus is created by means of a "flap". A flap is a term used in plastic surgery that refers to a piece of the patient's tissue that has a dedicated blood vessel that supplies and drains it with blood. This is needed so the tissue can survive and get nutrition and oxygen. In a phalloplasty this tissue usually constitutes skin, fat, and nerves in addition to the blood vessels. In the case of a belly-based flap, the donor site is tissue that is actually directly next to your future phallus position. Therefore, surgeons can just "fold" it down and leave the skin attached to its original location. The blood comes via those remaining skin attachments. If a patient is older or has health issues, a belly-based flap may be suggested as this option generally has fewer complications, a shorter surgery and hospital stay time. In case of a thigh flap the blood supply comes from a long artery and vein that usually does not need to be disconnected but can be "pedicled" or rotated to the phallus position. Pedicled means the flap is transferred with its original blood supply intact but will then be sutured at the base of the phallus to the final position.

In case of a "free flap" the blood supply is disconnected and then reconnected at the phallus position.

Options for phalloplasty donor sites include the forearm, thigh, lower belly, or back. Other donor sites such as the calf or upper arm have also been described but are rarely offered. At most institutions, forearm and thigh flaps are most commonly used, followed by belly-based flaps. Depending on the circumference of your forearm or the thickness of the skin of the thigh, one option may be more preferable than the other. A patient may be asked to lose weight to make a thigh-based option preferable. A patient may also be asked to lose wait to ensure the flap attachment to the recipient site is optimized for the greatest success. Previous surgeries or injuries that led to scarring may make a donor site not suitable. Depending on the donor site chosen, other work up can be necessary (e.g. computer tomogram of the leg to look at the blood vessels in the leg).

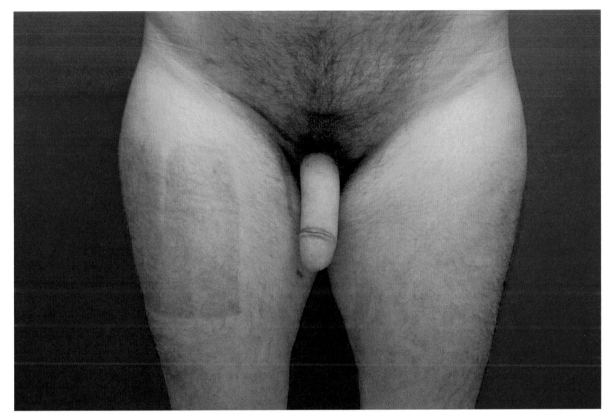

Figure 132 Phalloplasty from a radial free forearm flap - notice where skin grafts were taken from the tigh to cover the forearm.

Flap Design:

Depending on the donor site, the patient's anatomy (e.g. thickness of the flap), and the desired functional outcome there are three distinct ways the phallus is created.

A. Rectangular flap

In this option a rectangular flap is transferred where there is no inner tube. The tip is closed by means of a purse string suture. This type of design is typically used for a shaft-only phalloplasty without the ability to urinate from the tip. However, some surgeons use this design and then in subsequent surgeries "split" the phallus and create the urethra at a later stage (see staging below)

B. Tube Within tube

This is the most frequently used design for the forearm flaps (RFFFP) and in thin patients the thigh flap (ALT). In this technique the flap has two areas. One area that is a bit longer but only a ¼ of the width is used to create the urethra while the rest of the flap is used to create the shaft. This means the flap is rolled twice in opposite directions. At the end of the surgery there is skin facing inside and skin facing outside. The inner tube is the new urethra and will be connected to the part of the urethra that is created from your genital tissue (perineal urethra, pars fixa, urethral lengthening).

C. Composite Phalloplasty

In this option the shaft and neourethra are made from two flaps taken from separate sites on the body (e.g. thigh and lower belly). This type of phalloplasty is more complex and has a higher risk for complications. It is used if individuals are not a good candidate for a tube within tube phalloplasty.

Length/Girth

The length and diameter of the phallus are chosen to resemble an average erect penis of a cis male. The length can vary depending on preference and what your flap can offer, however ideal length is generally < 5.5 inches. The longer the phallus the more risk for complications, postvoid dribble and interference with physical activity. A phalloplasty is not attached to the pelvic bone, just the tissues overlying it. Therefore, it will stretch over the course of your lifetime. The heavier and larger a phallus the more it will stretch over the course of the next 10-50 years. This may require secondary surgeries to perform a "Phallus lift" or phallic shortening.

Multiple vs Single Stage

As if the above decisions were not already difficult enough there is another factor that you need to consider when deciding on a surgeon and that is in how many stages and with what techniques the surgery is performed. All surgeons will perform erectile and testicular implants at a separate surgery, but all other components may be combined differently.

The ways of staging are too different to give you a full overview. For example, some centers will perform a hysterectomy and vaginectomy at the same time in preparation for phalloplasty while most others perform a hysterectomy first (at least 3 months) before starting the phalloplasty. However, it is important for you to understand the staging options for the actual phalloplasty and urethral creation.

A. Single Stage

This means that both the perineal and shaft urethra are constructed in one surgery. The benefit is obvious that you only have to undergo two to three surgeries (hysterectomy, phalloplasty, implants).

B. Metoidioplasty First

Here the first surgery includes creation of a metoidioplasty with urethral lengthening. The scrotoplasty is performed in a different manner then a typical metoidioplasty but will be finalized at the secondary surgery. The benefit of this is that patients who are unsure can start out with this and if they are satisfied do not need to undergo further surgery. However, if urethral complications occur this may lead to an additional stage down the road.

C. Big Ben Method

In this method the shaft and shaft urethra are created first. The new urethra is left as an open end next to your clitoral shaft and will be connected to your native urethra at the second surgery. The benefit of this surgery is that the phallus can heal completely before the urinary system is connected. In case of complications with the flap, those can be dealt with separate from urine flowing through. Even the most severe complications (e.g. loss of the phallus) can be managed within the postoperative recovery. Since there is minimal surgery done to the genital region it is near fully reversible in case of grave complications.

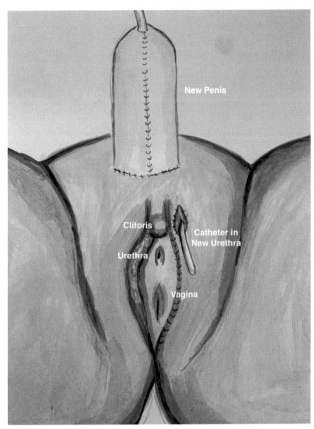

Figure 133 Big Ben method of creating phallus (urethra connected later).

D. Grafting Methods

This is a mixed bag of surgeries that all have one thing in common. They use "graft" material to create the shaft urethra. Graft is a piece of tissue that is very thin and does not have blood supply. Typically, it is taken from the mouth, skin, uterus, or vagina. Some surgeons "prelaminate it" – meaning they create a tube of graft within the future donor site. This is then transferred a few months later together with the shaft. Other surgeons do it after a shaft-only phalloplasty has been transferred by splitting the phallus and putting graft inside the phallus. This is then allowed to heal and in an additional surgery the split shaft is then closed over a catheter to create a neourethra.

The advantage of this is that it is non-hair bearing skin and also is thinner and allows to create a urethra even within a thicker thigh or back flap. The downside is that it does not have its own blood supply and therefor has a higher risk of contracting and possibly creating healing complications.

For considerations around glansplasty, scrotoplasty, erectile devices, and testicular implants see section "other surgeries"

Postoperative course

The postoperative course and care instructions are technique and surgeon-specific, and beyond what we can summarize in this chapter. It depends on what was done at each stage and how the patient handled the surgery. However here some general considerations in the postoperative period.

- After shaft creation the phallus will benefit from staying in an upright position for the duration of healing (roughly 4-6 weeks). Various strategies to achieve this are implemented by surgeons and patients.

- Some surgeons will limit the amount you can bend your hips for up to 4 weeks.

- Limit walking for 4-6 weeks after any genital surgery to let the small incisions heal without irritation.

- Good hygiene in the postoperative period is helpful in preventing infections.

- After urethral connection you can expect to have some form of catheter for up to 4-6 weeks. A suprapubic catheter is frequently used and is a direct catheter that goes through your lower belly into the bladder.

- Physical or occupational therapy can help in regaining strength and flexibility if an arm or leg is used as donor tissue. Physical therapy can also help regain strength in your pelvic floor following vaginectomy.

Sensation after surgery

During the surgery (except for belly-based flaps) the surgeons connect one of your clitoral nerves (and if more nerves are available one from your groin), to the nerves running in the flap. This is not like connecting a plug to an outlet – but rather those nerves will have to regrow, which is something that takes time. It can take well over a year for the final sensation outcome. You might have partial sensation, where some parts of the phallus have sensation, and some don't. Age and certain medications can make nerve regeneration slower.

Orgasm after surgery is almost always possible, but people have different experiences and some report that orgasm takes longer or feels different. A small percentage of patients may experience orgasm just from stimulating the phallus. The majority of patients will have to stimulate the buried clitoris to achieve orgasm. If you can easily and quickly have an orgasm now, you are more likely to

be able to orgasm after surgery. If you choose to have the clitoris buried as part of perineal masculinization, you will still be able to stimulate it indirectly.

The forearm donor site generally provides more sensation than the thigh donor site. The abdominal and back donor sites provide least sensation if any at all.

Other Surgeries

Glansplasty

During this surgery a skin graft is used to create a circumcised appearance of your phallus. It involves an oval incision about 1/3 up your phallus. The elevated skin and skin graft are used to create a ridge. In some patients this can flatten over time. If the ridge remains it can be used to apply an external erectile device.

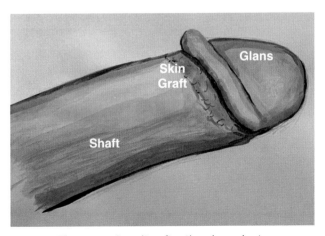

Figure 134 Results after the glansplasty.

Scrotoplasty/Testicular implants

See metoidioplasty section.

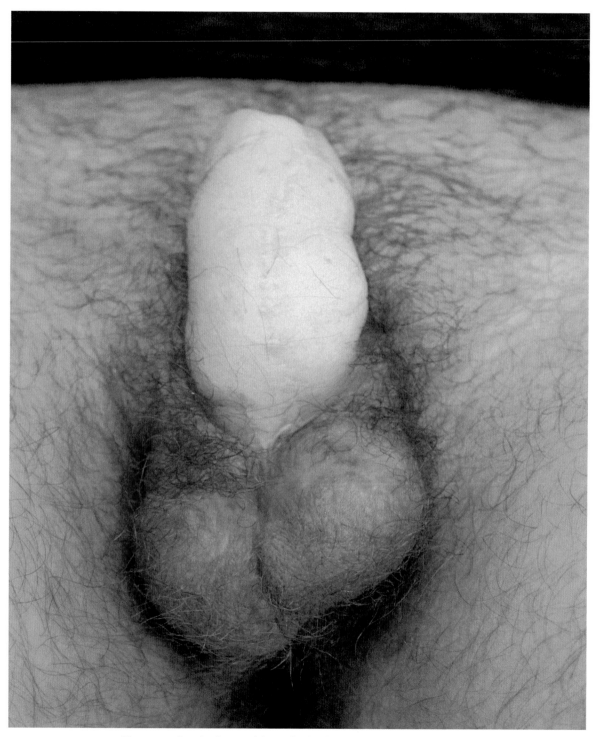

Figure 135Scrotoplasty with testicular implants after phalloplasty.

Secondary shaft revisions

The phallus can either have too much or too little girth. If it has too much, then the phallus can be thinned by either opening it up and cutting out fat and/or skin or by suctioning fat out through a small incision. If it is too thin, then fat can be injected that is taken from other parts of your body.

Erectile Implants

Some people decide to get a device implanted inside the phallus to create an erection. Due to the size and function of the metoidioplasty, internal erectile devices are only an option for phalloplasty patients.

There are two choices: the malleable device (a.k.a. semi-rigid rod) and the inflatable device.

Other people use external devices for an erection. Another option is the use of double condoms. There are also reports of using Coban (medical material used for splints) – we advise against that as it can prevent blood flow in and out of the phallus (e.g. falling asleep without removing it).

Cost and insurance coverage of these implants vary widely. Implants will not last a lifetime and will almost certainly need replacement or removal at some point.

Malleable device	Inflatable device
Lower cost	Higher cost
Easy to use, permanent semi-erection	Use fingers to use pump in the scrotum. Can be painful
Always the same semi-erect state.	Can change between flaccid (soft) or erect (hard) by pumping it
More visible through clothing and may be uncomfortable.	Less visible through clothing
Higher rate of extrusion through development of pressure sores	Higher rate of malfunction due to complex system with multiple small tubes. Possible higher rate of infection due to presence of more material.

Implanting a foreign body comes with potential complications such as:

- Injury to the blood supply of your phallus

- Injury to your urethra

- Infection

  - Antibiotics are typically given during surgery and for several days following surgery. Despite this, the infection rate following this surgery is still relatively high. If your implant gets infected, you will most likely have to have it removed. If possible, another implant can be inserted about a year later.

- Extrusion

  - This is from chronic pressure of the device on the inside of your phallus

  - It is important to deflate the device after use, and in case of semi-malleable devices to make sure the phallus is not pinched within your pants for too long (e.g. such as during air travel)

- Loosening from bony insertion (comes loose from where it is attached)

- Migration (the tip of the cylinders, scrotal pump, or other parts moving away from their intended location)

- Angle or strength (rigidity) if erection is insufficient

  - This can be due to the weight of your phallus, the angle of your pubic bone or other factors

  - In some cases, it is possible to revise the implant with two cylinders to improve rigidity

- Visible hardware through skin

- Chronic pain

- Failure of implant (breaks, or doesn't work anymore)

Risks & Complications

The metoidioplasty and phalloplasty processes are long. They will likely include multiple stages, and several regions on the body are affected. While your surgeon will do their best to avoid complications, they can and do arise with varying severity. Complications can change the course, so having a flexible mindset in the postoperative period is key to addressing issues healthfully, if they arise. Surgeons who offer these procedures routinely will be able to manage most complications successfully, but it may mean additional surgery and longer recovery. Below we have outlined common risks and complications associated with metoidioplasty and phalloplasty, keep in mind that this does not replace an in-depth conversation with your surgeon and that this is an incomplete list that only mentions the most frequent.

This following list includes only the most frequent types of complications.

General Surgical Risks:

Pain

Pain following surgery is inevitable and everyone's pain experience is different. Patients experience different levels of pain, different types of pain, and for varying lengths of time. Patient's may report pain at some surgical areas and none at others. While most pain subsides over the first 4-6 weeks following each stage, minor discomfort or pain is normal even beyond the normal healing period and usually subsides within a year after surgery. While rare it is possible for patients to have long-term pain or "chronic pain". Another source of pain can be the cut nerve endings in the groin, arm or leg

that form a "neuroma" – which is an irritated nerve ending and can be treated through repeat surgery.

Wound separation – This is one of the more common complications after surgery. Wound separation happens in places where two areas of skin have been stitched together but the skin edges pull apart after surgery. Wound separation typically heals on its own with keeping the site clean and dry and performing regular dressing changes. It is also important to limit walking during the healing period as friction can increase the risk for wound separation. Open wounds heal on their own but can sometimes form granulation tissue or fibrin. Fibrin is a white substance and may be mistaken for pus. Open wounds however rarely get infected and your surgeon can tell you what it is.

Granulation tissue – This is an area of bright red/pink tissue around an incision where healing wasn't complete. Some people call this "proud flesh" and it is essentially the body creating too much tissue when trying to heal. It can sometimes present as painless bleeding or spotting at the surgical site. This is also quite common and can be treated with silver nitrate (or chemical small burn) at follow-up visits.

Tissue necrosis - or "tissue death", occurs when there is a lack of blood flow to healing tissues. This is an uncommon problem. Depending on the location and severity, a "wait-and-see" approach may be used, with regular dressing changes. If the tissue needs repair, this would require a second revision surgery.

Regret – Regret is a very complex and difficult topic. Reasons for regret are vary widely. A temporary degree of regret early after surgery is not uncommon. Complications can also lead to regret and it is therefore really important that you understand all the potential risks and understand how they may affect your life. Similarly, outcomes vary depending on your anatomy so make sure to ask your surgeon what you can and cannot expect. Any limitations that you accept preoperatively will not lead to disappointment. However, if you only find out after the surgery that your result may not be as hoped then this can cause significant distress. This type of regret is a particular concern for metoidioplasty. Even if it is a goal and the plan is the ability to stand and urinate it may not be possible.

Similarly, the results are often not as visible to the patients, especially if there is significant weight gain later in life. Many patients have seen ideal results of other folks' surgeries online and hope to have the same result. But everyone's anatomy is different, and no two surgical results are the same (even with the same surgeon).

True regret of having undergone surgical transition is fortunately exceedingly rare however also a reality that few individuals may experience.

Infection – Signs of infection generally include spreading redness, pus discharge, odor, swelling, warmth to touch, red streaking, or fever. If you have concern for infection, you should contact your surgeon immediately.

If you have diabetes, be sure to take extra care and be diligent about checking and correcting your blood sugar – because the stress of surgery can make it more difficult to control blood sugar. Poorly controlled blood sugar increases a diabetic's risk of infection.

Hematoma – This is localized bleeding outside of blood vessels. If you develop a sudden, swelling and/or significant bruising at the surgical site, you may have a hematoma. Small hematomas typically resolve on their own. Large hematomas may need to be drained.

Blood clots (sudden leg swelling and/or pain or difficulty breathing)
– Blood clots in your veins can form during and after surgery due to prolonged inactivity. If you notice that one of your legs swells suddenly or starts hurting, or if you suddenly have a hard time breathing – then you may have a blood clot. You should go to the Emergency Department immediately.

Urinary Complications:

Urinary spray

When patients begin urinating from their neourethra, they can experience irregular urinary stream or spray. This makes standing urination challenging. Urinary spray can improve over several months as the surgical sites heal but can also be an ongoing issue. Your surgeon may be able to address this issue by adjusting the urethral opening.

Fistula

A fistula is a type of wound healing issue that results in an unwanted open connection between two regions. In the case of phalloplasty, fistulas appear in the setting of an unwanted opening between the outside world and the neourethra which causes urinary leakage. Fistulas sometime heal on their own but if they fail to do so then an outpatient surgery to close that fistula is needed. This often requires a urinary catheter for a short duration of time (<14 days)

Urinary Stricture – A stricture is narrowing of the urethra and can occur in areas of scarring or trauma. If patients notice a weak urine stream, have a feeling like they aren't fully emptying their bladder, have more frequent urination, or have an inability to pee altogether, then they may have a stricture. If you can't urinate then an emergent placement of a catheter is needed. Usually a suprapubic catheter is used to redirect the urine. Subsequent surgery is needed to release the narrowing and can involve one or more surgeries.

Urine retention/ Difficulty emptying bladder – Rarely people notice that it is difficult to empty the bladder after having the suprapubic catheter removed. If this happens, we would likely perform diagnostic tests to determine what the problem is and/

or replace the catheter to drain your bladder

Post void dribble

Post void dribble is a very common finding following phalloplasty with urethral lengthening. This is when a patient experiences a small amount of urine in the neourethra following urination, such that the moments following urination they may notice some urine dribble from the phallus. This is a difficult issue to treat surgically, however the patient can help remove the retained urine by gently pressing along the outside of the urethra (milking).

Urinary urgency/frequency – This is a feeling of having to pee suddenly and often. This is common soon after surgery due to bladder irritation. This typically resolves on its own.

Bladder and rectal injury are rare but serious complications. Accidental injury to the bladder or rectum can occur during vaginectomy. If we identify this early, it can be repaired during surgery. If we do not identify the injury, other complications may arise and another surgery will be required to fix this.

Graft failure – Buccal Graft:
For metoidioplasty with urethral lengthening, we use a skin graft from your inner cheek to help lengthen your urethra. Total graft failure is rare. More often than not, small areas of the graft may fail, and this would typically resolve on its own or with non-surgical intervention. It may also result in urethral fistula or stricture, which are discussed further down.

Flap and Donor Site Complications

Flap loss

This occurs when all or part of the flap dies due to poor blood flow. Total flap loss is rare but is a risk that patients should know about. If part of the flap dies, the affected portion can be removed by your surgeon and the phallus can be reconstructed immediately or at a later date. Flap loss is most common during the first few weeks after surgery, and therefore proper phallus position and body position is vital during this time to ensure the best possible blood flow to the phallus.

Arm or Leg weakness/stiffness

Due to the amount of tissue taken from the thigh and forearm to create the phallus, it is possible for one to experience weakness or decreased flexibility in the affected hand/ forearm or leg. Hand therapy and physical therapy can help a patient regain strength and range of motion to a near-normal state, but permanent weakness is possible.

Skin graft failure: The flap donor site (forearm or thigh) are covered with a thin layer of skin that is taken from the thigh (opposite thigh if using a thigh-based flap). This skin will survive by adhering and getting oxygen from the wound bed underneath. If the graft does not attach, then some areas may not survive and need to be removed. Small areas will fill in by wound healing over time. If a large area is lost, a repeat skin graft may be needed to cover the region.

4. Facial Masculinization Surgery

By Dr. Barry Eppley

Facial masculinization surgery (FMS) refers to a collection of aesthetic surgeries aimed at making various facial features appear more masculine. This typically means making the eight (8) facial bony points more prominent. These include the brows, cheeks, nose, chin and jaw angles. Like **facial feminization surgery** (FFS), these surgeries are often associated with transgender patients. But FMS is more frequently sought out by cisgender men seeking stronger and more defined facial features. It is the experience from these more commonly done facial masculinization surgeries that translates to the female to male transgender patient.

While FFS surgery has many reductive procedures to achieve its effects, facial masculinization is the converse...many of the needed procedures involve some form of bone augmentation to create the facial angularity and definition that is perceived as being more masculine. While there are numerous FMS procedures available, and most patients do not choose or need to undergo all of them, it's extremely common to undergo more than one procedure in a surgery to get the best transformative (or enhancing) effect.

Preoperative Evaluation

The preoperative FMS process allows the doctor and patient to get on the same page in terms of goals and treatment options. Considering that many of the procedures performed as part of facial reshaping surgery create potentially irreversible changes, it is essential that patients are aware and have input into the flavor of facial change that these procedures create. As such, preoperative computer imaging helps better set the facial reshaping goals and manage patient expectation. No patient should undergo FMS without some sort of predictive tool aiding the decision process. Although computer imaging is an essential component of the preoperative process, it's merely representative of an approximation of the facial changes that may occur. Its best benefit is in creating a visual means of communication in what is otherwise a very individual and somewhat abstract concept. (what looks good one my face?)

Facial Masculinization Surgery Procedures

Facial masculinization procedures are broken down into four categories based on the associated zones of treatment: skull/forehead, midface, lower jaw and neck. Despite the number of facial procedures performed or the facial zones treated, FMS is almost always done in an outpatient surgery center under general anesthesia. Surgery time may be as little as one hour or it may take considerably longer for more complete cases with multiple procedures. For the longer surgery procedures, it may be necessary to stay overnight for the immediate recovery.

FOREHEAD/SKULL *(Upper Third)*

In this section the art of surgical masculinization of the upper third of the face will discuss the role of the following two procedures:

1) Brow bone augmentation

2) Forehead augmentation

3) Forehead-Brow Bone Augmentation

4) Temporal Augmentation

5) Skull Augmentation

Brow Bone Augmentation

Brow bone prominences with a suprabrow bone break are the hallmark of a masculine upper third of the face. Men always have some semblance of brow bone prominences while the vast majority of women do not. In the past, the typical surgical approach has been the application of bone cements or a handmade implant material through an open coronal scalp incision placed behind the hairline. This approach is fraught with potential brow bone shape/irregularity issues not to mention the long scalp scar needed to place them. I now consider this an historic approach with significant aesthetic liabilities.

The contemporary and far more effective technique is to use a custom brow bone implant made from the patient's 3D CT scan. The presurgical design process allows for the exact amount of increased brow bone prominence, its shape and complex topography across the glabellar area as well as how far it extends down along the lateral orbital rim. While it may appear on a cursory glance that the brow bone is a horizontal straight bar of bone across the top of the eyes, this is far too simplistic design approach. It actually has one of the most complex 3D shapes of any bone on the face due primarily to the frontal sinus cavities which comprise the central region. Getting the 'eagle wing' shape of the brow bones and transitioning that into the lateral brow is an art form onto itself.

The brow bone implant can be placed using an endoscopic approach through a small scalp incision which may or may not need to be aided by small lateral upper eyelid incisions (depending upon how far down along the lateral orbital rims the implant design goes).

Such brow bone implants can be done alone if one has an adequate forehead shape above it.

Forehead Augmentation

The shape of the male forehead is less rounded and vertically inclined than that of the female. For the female to male patient the vertical inclination of the forehead may be satisfactory, but it may have inadequate width and lack a slightly flatter/broader/shape. This really has to do with the location of the bony temporal lines which are the lateral transition points of the bony forehead to the soft tissue temporal area. Women typically lack them due to their convex forehead shapes while their presence in men is more visible. Besides the presence of brow bones this is a defining feature of the male forehead.

Creating a more masculine forehead shape involves broadening the bony lateral borders of the forehead over onto the temporalis fascia to create the needed width. When the shape change is combined with the large surface area of the forehead and creates a completely smooth surface, the best approach is a custom forehead implant design. This also has the added advantage of a much smaller scalp incision for placement. Bone cements can be used but they require a more open approach with longer scalp incisions and rely on the intraoperative artistic shaping of a moldable bone cement material.

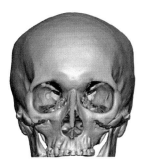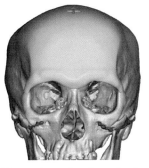

Figure 136 Custom forehead brow-bone implant design

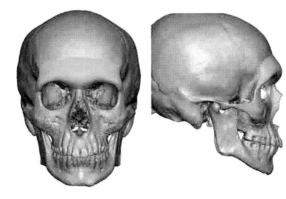

Figure 137 Custom Forehead Implant design

Forehead-Brow Bone Augmentation

Depending upon how deficient the upper third of the face is, a combined forehead-brow bone implant may be beneficial. This has the most transformative effect as it completely changes the shape of the forehead in a controlled manner in a single implant design. It is the only facial reshaping procedure in which a third of the face is altered in its entirety by one single implant.

Temporal Augmentation

While the natural shape of the temples is slightly concave in both genders, females tend to have increased temporal concavities. Temporal concavities or hollowing are measured by making a straight line from the lateral bony temporal line of the forehead down to the zygomatic arch. The depth of the temporal skin below this line in its midportion is the depth of the temporal concavity. Men typically prefer an almost straighter temporal surface shape. This is also more aesthetically pleasing and compatible with a broader forehead shape.

Temporal augmentation can be done with fillers, fat and implants. While temporary injectable fillers can help with making a reversible decision about any change, the debate in permanent augmentation really comes down to fat injections vs implants. That decision is guided by the magnitude of the change desired and its priority level in the overall facial reshaping efforts. If only a modest augmentation is needed fat injections, despite their unpredictable volume retention, is an appropriate match for the level of concern. More significant and assured augmentation comes from the use of standard temporal implants which are designed to augment the entire non-hair bearing temporal area. (anterior temporal zone) These are muscle augmentation implants that are placed underneath the temporal fascia from an incision behind the ear and typically cover from the zygomatic arch up to, but just below, the lateral temporal line. Because they do not cross the temporal line this will not have a forehead widening effect

For the more narrow head, which refers to the temporal region in the hair-bearing scalp along the side of the head (posterior temporal zone), temporal augmentation can be done to create an enhanced head width effect. Using a custom temporal implant design, which is also introduced from an incision behind the ear, the implant is placed either under the temporal muscle or underneath the temporal fascia on top of the muscle. (based on the extent of the implant coverage) Such posterior temporal augmentations can very effectively increase head width/ convexity.

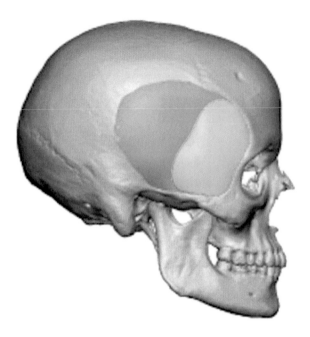

Figure 138 Extended anterior temporal implant design

Skull Augmentation

There a number of features of the skull that are more commonly associated with men than women. While most of these recognized differences are in the forehead, the male skull tends to be both thicker and broader. This creates a head shape that is wider between the temporal lines with a less convex top of the head shape in the frontal view. The width of the sides of the head is also greater, or at least has greater convexity due to a thicker temporal muscle.

Besides the capability to increase the width of the head through temporal augmentation, the shape of the top of the head can be altered as well through the use of custom skull implant designs. The head can be made broader with less convexity and have more visible temporal lines if desired. Placed through a small scalp incision as compared to the width of the implant, substantial skull shape modifications can be reliably achieved.

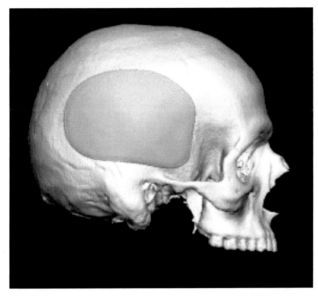

Figure 139 Custom head widening temporal implant

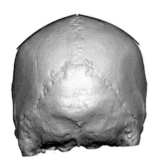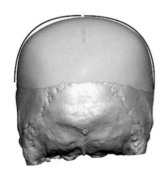

Figure 140 Custom masculinizing skull implants back view

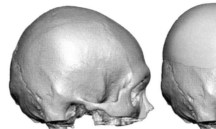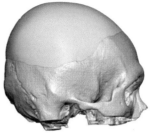

Figure 141 Custom masculinizing skull implant design side view

MIDFACE *(Middle Third)*

In this section the art of reshaping of the middle third of the face to a more masculine appearance we will discuss the role of the following procedures:

6) Rhinoplasty

7) Cheek Augmentation

8) Infraorbital Augmentation

9) Buccal Lipectomies and Perioral Liposuction

Rhinoplasty

Rhinoplasty is a common facial masculinization procedure given that there are major gender differences in the shape of the nose. A masculine nose typically has a straight or even slightly convex dorsal line in side profile. It also has a nasal tip that is not overly narrow and a nasolabial angle that is at 95 degrees or less. Some artists even describe the male nose as being sharper and more chiseled in shape. (works well in drawings and caricature rendering, not so sure that translates to a surgical goal) To achieve these changes in a nose that has distinctly feminine characteristics requires dorsal augmentation and tip derotation/lengthening. In some cases, a wider bridge or tip area may also be desired.

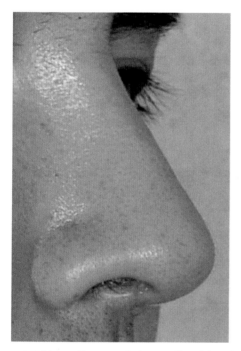

Figure 142 Masculine nasal shape after rhinoplasty

If the only nasal change needed is to increase the height of the bridge, this can be done through a variety of dorsal augmentation techniques. The debate is always which augmentation method is to be used which comes down to a cartilage graft (usually rib) vs an implant. Each has their advantages and disadvantages which are well known and both techniques can be very effective. Rib grafts have the benefits of not being an implant but shaping it and preventing it from warping after surgery are its challenges. Dicing the rib graft and wrapping it in fascia overcomes these issues. Implants have the advantage of not having to be harvested and come with an assured shape. The key with implants in the nose is to use an implant layered or totally made of ePTFE (expanded polytetrafluroethylene). This material allows for tissue adherence and has less risk of complications in the nose than a pure silicone implant.

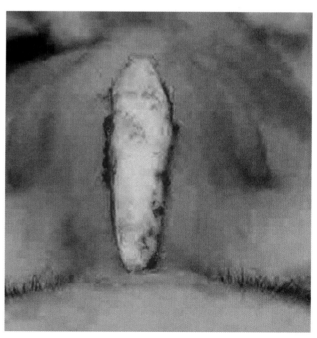

Figure 143 Rib graft during surgery

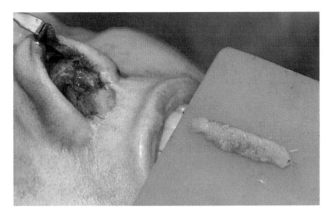

Figure 144 Diced rib graft rhinoplasty

nasal airflow if needed. If the combination of dorsal augmentation and tip lengthening/derotation are the rhinoplasty changes needed, then the volume of graft supplied by rib cartilage is needed.

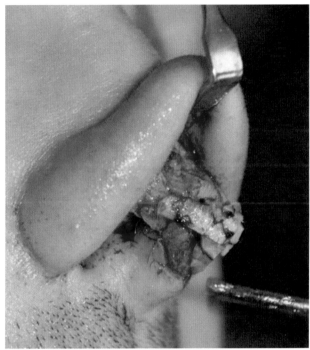

Figure 146 Tip lengthening and derotation in masculinizing rhinoplasty

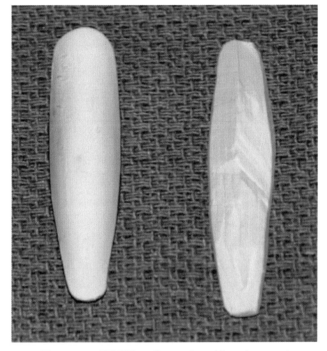

Figure 145 EPTFE preformed and hand carved nasal implants

Controlled changes in the tip of the nose require cartilage grafts for bringing the tip down (derotation) as well as to widen it if needed. Such cartilage grafts are usually harvested from the septum where concurrent septal straightening/inferior turbinate reduction can be done to improve

Cheek Augmentation

Male cheeks typically have more fullness higher on the main body of the cheek bone (zygoma) and back along the tail of the cheekbone (zygomatic arch) for more defined and angular cheek highlights. Standard styles of cheek implants are usually not sufficient in FMS as their creation of an 'apple cheek' look is associated with a feminine midface. Custom designed cheek implants are used to create this uniquely 'high cheekbone' look that better suits the male face. As part of the high cheekbone look the infraorbital (under eye) area is often included in the design as well. Placed through a lower eyelid incision the implant creates a line of midface augmentation from under the eye, around the corner of the cheek and back along the zygomatic arch.

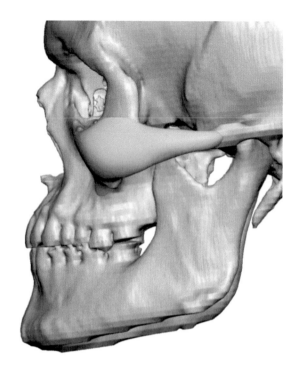

Figure 148 Male custom high cheek bone implants side view

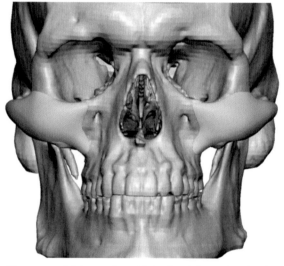

Figure 147 Male custom high cheek bone implants

There is a role for fat injections in male cheek augmentation but less so than in female cheeks. Fat usually produces a softer or rounder type of cheek appearance which is more distinctly feminine. This can be avoided by using more of a straight-line placement approach to create more of a linear augmentation effect.

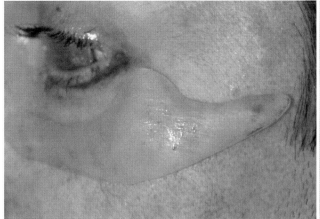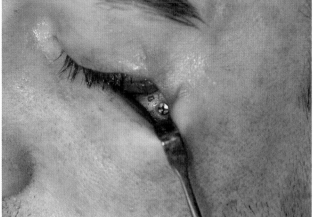

Figure 149 Hemi-lid incision for custom infra-orbital malar implants

Buccal Lipectomies and Perioral Mound Liposuction

Most men desire a more angular facial shape. To achieve this (or to de-round the face) as much as possible, the removal of selective areas of facial fat can complement other facial augmentation procedures. Besides the neck, the only areas of the face where fat can be removed is the buccal pads and subcutaneous fat around the mouth and back along the jawline. These select areas of fat can be removed via small incisions inside the mouth with buccal lipectomy and perioral mound/jawline microliposuction techniques. Such facial fat removal has a modest, not a dramatic, reductive facial contouring effect between the bony cheeks and

bony jawline. This is why they are usually done in conjunction with other facial augmentation procedures to create a complementary effect rather than just being done alone.

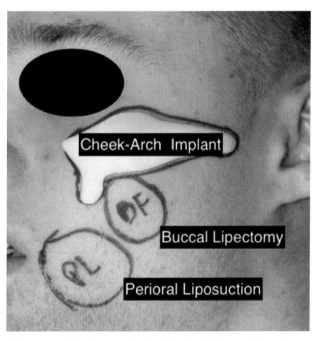

Figure 150 Custom malar implant with buccal lipectomy and perioral liposuction

LOWER FACE (Lower Third)

In this section the art of masculine reshaping of the lower third of the face will discuss the role of the following procedures:

10) Chin Implants

11) Sliding Geniplasty

12) Jaw Angle Implants

13) Custom Jawline Implant

14) Tracheal Augmentation

15) Neck Liposuction/ Submentoplasty

Chin Augmentation

Chin augmentation is the single most important lower-face procedure in FMS. (A prominent chin is a wholly distinct male feature) Chin augmentation is often perceived only in the profile, ignoring the appearance from the front view. So, it is important to consider the appearance of the chin from the front view, assessing the chin width and squareness as well. An augmented chin that appears more masculine often has a squarer shape to it.

Chin augmentation is usually done by an implant which has the aesthetic advantages of creating increased horizontal projection and width/ squareness as well. There are multiple materials from which chin implants are made but solid silicone has the greatest number of styles and sizes and is the easiest to surgically place. (and remove/modify if desired) Chin implants can be introduced through an intraoral or submental skin incision. The submental approach is associated with a lower risk of infection and implant malpositioning.

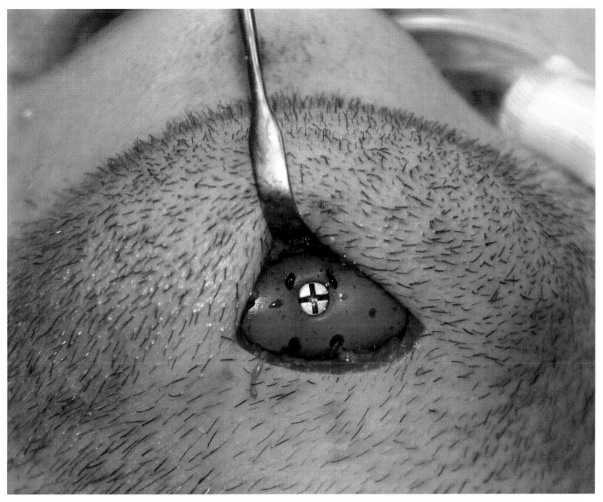

Figure 151 Chin implant screwed into position

Sliding Genioplasty

The cousin to the chin implant is the sliding genioplasty. It has the aesthetic advantage of providing a horizontal as well as a vertical projection increase if desired, so called 45-degree chin augmentation effect. It is often preferred by patients who need larger amounts of chin projection and/or are opposed to having an implant material in their face. The one aesthetic disadvantage to the sliding genioplasty is that it cannot make the chin wider or more square. (and in significant increase in horizontal projection may make it look more narrow) This disadvantage can be overcome by using a chin implant overlay placed on the front edge of the sliding genioplasty to create this missing dimensional change.

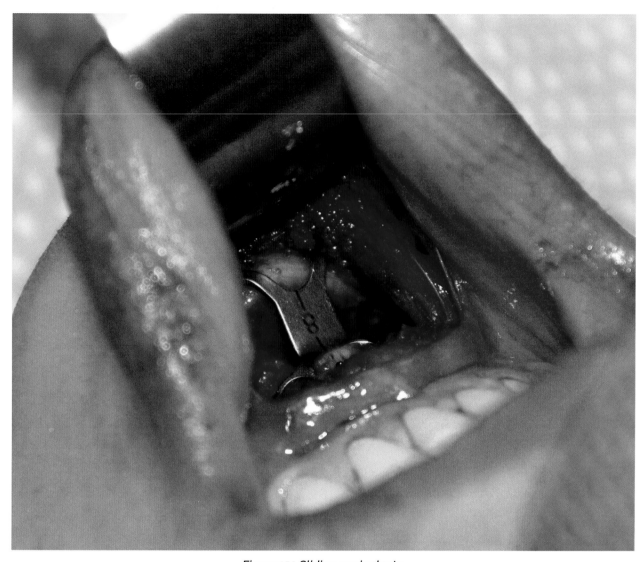

Figure 152 Sliding genioplasty

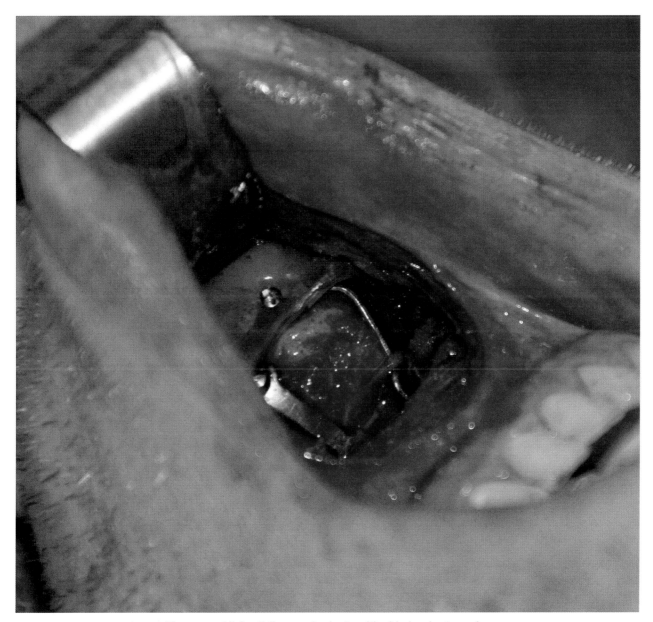

Figure 153 Male sliding genioplasty with chin implant overlay

Jaw Angle Implants

Besides the chin the other key feature of the male lower face is the jawline. Patients often refer to wanting their jawline enhanced and the surgeon immediately assumes this will be solved by a chin augmentation. What the patient is actually referring to with the word 'jawline' is the jaw angle area or a combination of both the chin and jaw angles. This means the entire jawline from the chin to the jaw angles. Having more defined jaw angles together with a prominent chin creates a lower third of the face that defines masculinity.

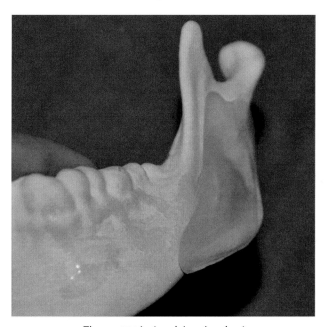

Figure 154 Lateral Jaw Implant

The traditional approach to achieving this total jawline effect is

with standard chin and jaw angles implants. Jaw angle implants are placed through intraoral incisions underneath the masseter muscle. They are either placed directly over the perimeter of the bony jaw angles (widening jaw angle implants) or a portion of the implant lies behind the existing bony jaw angle border (vertical lengthening jaw angle implants).

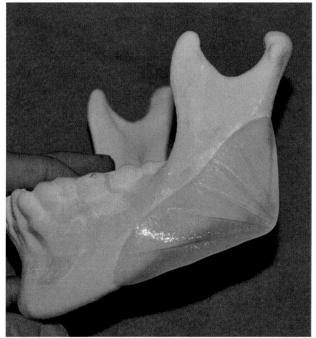

Figure 155 Vertical Lengthening Jaw angle implant

Total Jawline Augmentation

While standard chin and jaw angle implants can work well for many jawline augmentation patients, they lack a linear connection between the three corners of the jaw augmentations. (chin and jaw angles) To overcome this potential aesthetic deficiency and create the most profound lower jaw augmentation effect is the custom jawline implant, also known as a jaw wraparound implant.

In a circumferential manner along the entire lower border of the lower

jaw an implant can be designed to change its entire shape. Both size and angularity can be created in a 3D fashion. Placed through a three incision technique (submental skin with paired intraoral incisions) the one-piece implant can be inserted and secured.

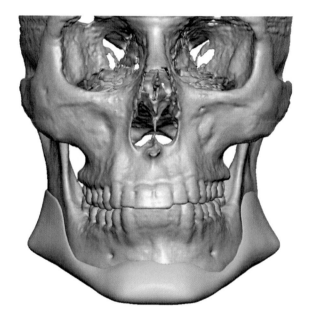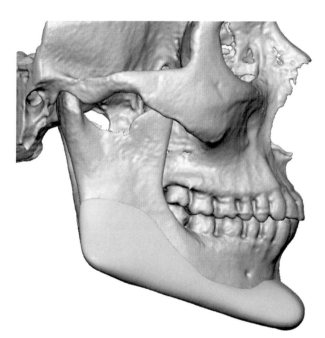

Figure 156 Custom Jawline Implant

Tracheal Augmentation

A prominent Adam's apple or thyroid cartilage creates a central neck bulge that is a distinctively male trait. Its reduction, of course, is the one of the most well-known facial feminization procedures. Conversely the trachea can be augmented in

the FMS patient by a special implant designed to create a more prominent v-shaped thyroid notch prominence. The tracheal augmentation implant is placed through a small overlying skin incision identical to that used in a tracheal shave procedure. The implant is placed on top of the existing thyroid cartilage and secured with sutures. It is made of a material that permits tissue ingrowth that adds to its assured long-term positional stability.

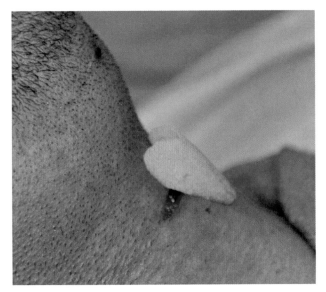

Figure 157 Male tracheal implant

Liposuction/Submentoplasty

To help make for a more visible chin and/or jawline, defatting of the fat beneath them may have an additive effect. This can be done either by liposuction or with central platysma muscle tightening as well. (submentoplasty) A submentoplasty is a graduated procedure over liposuction which is often overlooked in neck reshaping. By adding muscle tightening (and submuscular defatting) with liposuction the greatest improvement in the cervicomental angle can be obtained.

Facial Masculinization Surgery Recovery

The FMS recovery process largely revolves around the amount of swelling that occurs during treatment. Fortunately, the swelling is more of an aesthetic issue rather than a functional issue, meaning that patients recovering from FMS shouldn't experience any functional limitations.

The amount of swelling that occurs is largely down to the type and number of procedures performed. That said, there are general postoperative guidelines that can help to estimate the amount of swelling to expect after treatment. Approximately 50 percent of facial swelling should subside within 10 to 14 days after surgery. Close to 65 percent should subside within three weeks of treatment, and virtually all swelling of significance should be gone by six weeks after surgery. But the final results of the surgery cannot be fully assessed until at least three months after surgery, at which point swelling has subsided *and* the overlying soft tissues have contracted back down over the augmented facial framework.

As one gets through the early recovery phase from FMS, it is important to point out that one's initial concerns are largely going to be the opposite of FFS. In reductive FFS one is focused on whether the face has been reduced enough and the early swelling makes one feel that it is still too big in many areas. In augmentative FMS, one will feel early on that the face is too big and has been over corrected.

Complications and Risks

FMS procedures are generally very safe with high success rates. However, as with any medical procedure, there is the potential for complications. Because MFS often uses implants to create the desired changes, this makes the most significant medical risks that of infection and permanent numbness of nerves close to the implanted facial areas. Fortunately, these complications are not common.

The aesthetic risks of FMS surgery are usually of greater relevance and are how the facial outcome appears and how it is perceived by the patient. For example, augmentative changes may be more (or less) pronounced than expected. As a result, there is always the risk of the need for revision of the

procedures to optimize their aesthetic outcomes.

Facial Masculinization Surgery Cost & Insurance Coverage

The only way to get an accurate assessment of the cost of FMS is to schedule a virtual consultation and have your pictures assessed and imaged. The cost can vary greatly depending on the number of procedures performed, the cost of the implants used (if any), the operative time required for the surgery, and the location at which it is performed.

The cost of FMS may be covered by insurance in cases of documented female-to-male transgender surgery. However, for the more common instances of men seeking to improve their natural genetic appearance, the treatment is viewed as purely cosmetic and therefore not covered.

Consult a Qualified MFS Surgeon

Here are some tips to consider when consulting a surgeon about MFS:

- Create a list of the facial changes you think would be most helpful for the best transformation to discuss with your surgeon. This will help the surgeon understand your expectations and develop a treatment plan.

- Ask where the surgery will be performed, the extent of the procedure and whether it is going to be done as an outpatient or overnight stay.

- Ask about complications and possible side effects of the procedure (they can and do happen).

Ask the recovery period and your activities after surgery so you can plan properly for the time needed.

5. Hair Loss and Skin Care

By Dr. Sidhbh Gallagher

Managing Baldness

Androgenetic Alopecia

One of the known side effects of taking testosterone is baldness or the medical term for this is androgenic alopecia. It's not known exactly how common this is, but in one study 43% of transmen, and 35% of nonbinary individuals reported scalp hair loss or thinning.

Why some patients on testosterone develop baldness and others don't is down to how the body and hair follicles respond to testosterone. Genes largely predict that. Taking a look at how common baldness is in your family will give you a big clue as to whether you may develop it on testosterone.

While this of course may not bother some patients, options are needed for folks it does bother.

Some patients may choose to come off testosterone altogether- a discussion needs to be had with your hormone provider before doing this. This is especially true if the ovaries have been removed as, depending on the patient's age, probably some sort of hormones are needed to continue to be healthy.

There are however other options.

Minoxidil

This is a topical treatment such as a shampoo so there are less concerns about interfering with hormone levels. It comes in either 2% or 5% solutions and is often used twice a day. Unfortunately, it requires continuous use and only about a third of patients see real results. These numbers are from cis-gender men – the studies still need to be done for transgender men.

Finasteride

This medication, again, isn't widely studied in transgender men, however a small study showed good results and no side effects.

The concern with this medication is it may counteract the changes we want to see on testosterone. Ideally therefore, it shouldn't be used while these changes are still developing (such as lowering of the voice or bottom growth) in the first couple of years.

Interestingly hair loss on the temples isn't improved but the hairline and the "bald spot" on the top of the head may be improved.

Other options

Different types Lasers have been used with some positive results however more studies are needed.

Surgery or "hair plugs" can be very effective because the technique borrows hairs from areas not effected so much by testosterone (back of the scalp) and transplants it to where it's needed such as the hairline at the front.

Your Skin on Testosterone

Gradually, being on testosterone can drastically change a patient's skin.

Pores become larger, the skin itself may become thicker and the skin produces more sebum and sweat.

Two main unwanted side effects may result from these changes- the skin may appear to age faster and of course patient can develop acne.

Aging

For the first issue there is a massive industry based on antiaging treatments for the skin. Firstly, a good antiaging skincare routine is needed, as described in the other chapter on skin care. Sunscreen is a must year-round and smoking needs to be avoided. Botox, fillers and resurfacing may be also be useful.

Acne

Acne is a very common unwanted side effect of testosterone.

One study showed it developed in 9% of the transgender men after 3 months and in 18% after 6 months. After 2 years, 38% of the transgender men had developed acne at some point. In that study risk factors for developing acne were patients with a higher BMI and smokers. Patients with higher testosterone levels were more likely to develop acne also.

Treatment

When treating acne, we want to control outbreaks and prevent scarring. First patients should try over the counter treatments, however something stronger may be needed if there is no change after a few weeks. Also, it may be appropriate to recheck hormone levels to make sure the testosterone level is not too high. It's known that levels over 630 ng/dL are more likely to lead to acne.

Both topical medications and medications taken by mouth can be given.

Common topical medications include:

- Antibiotics such as clindamycin or erythromycin usually taken along with benzoyl peroxide in order decrease bacterial counts.

- Retinoids can help decrease follicle plugging.

- Salicylic acid and azelaic acid- these can help prevent follicle clogging and are often used in combination with antibiotics.

Medications by mouth:

- In more severe cases the antibiotic may be better given by mouth – usually doxycycline is prescribed for as short a time as possible to control the acne and prevent resistance.

- Isoretinoin is a powerful medication but is only used in severe cases as it can have serious side effects such as depression and suicide.

Other treatments

These can include various lasers and chemical peels. Also, sometimes a steroid injected into a red inflamed spot may cause rapid relief.

Life after Surgery

By Dr. Sidhbh Gallagher

It is important to think ahead about life back home after surgery and how things will be as a patient slowly returns to their routine.

For many it is a happy time, feeling relieved and accomplished but this is not, by any means the rule and some patients will experience real depression.

It is good to be prepared for this in case it happens.

Other patients may feel a little lost for a time as they have spent so long working towards surgery now that goal is accomplished, they will need a new one.

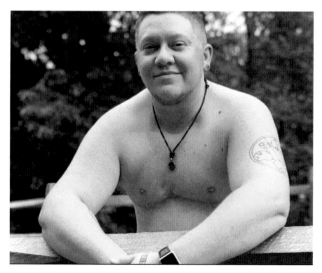

Figure 158 Patient after Masculoplasty.

Depression after Surgery.

We see it very regularly in the days and weeks after surgery, and sometimes it is so overwhelming that patients attempt to take their own lives. It is something you must watch out for, and be ready for, and have a plan in case it happens to you.

Why does it happen?

It seems counter intuitive! So many people are so excited about their gender confirmation surgery. They've worked so hard, to get here and finally the day arrives, all goes well with the surgery, they are recovering physically well afterwards, but are feeling terribly low, and why is that?

These are some of the reasons I believe why patients struggle with depression after surgery;

1. **Pain.** There are a lot of real physiological things going on. Surgery is a massive stressor; in that you are dealing with pain. We try to do everything we can to make our patients as comfortable as possible, but unfortunately pain

will always be there, hopefully not too overwhelming.

2. **Hormones.** Around the time of surgery, depending on what surgery you have, you can have a massive fluctuation in your hormones. For example, for our MTF bottom surgery patients, we have them hold off their hormones before surgery to prevent blood clots and then at the time of surgery, again if they are having testicles removed, we can see huge swings in these hormone levels. This results in patients feeling tired, lousy and tearful.

3. **Loss of daily routine.** Also you are away from the familiarity of your daily routine and find yourself in alien surroundings, instead of enjoying a coffee in the work canteen you are sitting in a hospital bed, you are not seeing your usual social contacts only unfamiliar people and all this can be very upsetting.

4. **Permanence Anxiety.** There is always going to be an element of permanence anxiety, this overwhelming feeling of "what have I done to myself". This, from what my patients tell me, is pretty much the norm and can last quite a long time as well. This is not necessarily regret but just a scary feeling that goes with all these new unfamiliar routines and changes in your anatomy.

What is clear from all of the above is that a plan is needed for after surgery. This may be a quick and easy way to check in with your therapist, if you are beginning to feel overwhelmed, or at least knowing that your support system is there.

This is a serious issue but know that it is temporary, know that it is quite a normal part of recovery for a lot of patients.

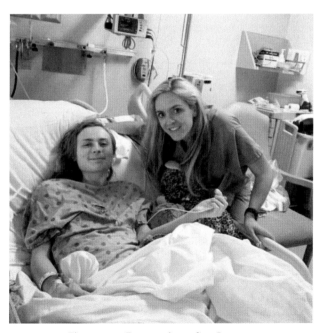

Figure 159 Recovering after Surgery

Life after recovery

Anatomy Inventory

One thing a patient must be clear on as they move on with their lives is their "anatomy inventory". This means just knowing what parts of the anatomy are still present. For example, in the case of a transfeminine patient after bottom surgery she will more than likely still have her prostate or does a transmasculine patient have a cervix still?

One important reason to know is if you have it, it needs to be checked as usual as part of a physical – be it an examination, a mammogram or a pap.

Unfortunately, as yet not all doctors fully understand the specific needs of the transgender population, so it is advisable that the patients know their parts!

Sexual health must also be kept in mind. STDs are very possible in the new anatomy so patients should be screened accordingly.

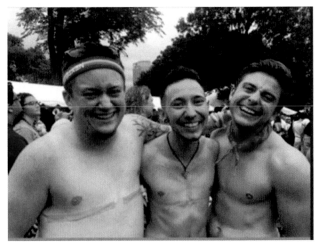

Figure 160 Many of my patients have wonderful support systems - here three masculoplasty patients celebrate pride.

What is Next?

Surgery isn't usually the "end" of transitioning. For many it's an on-going sometimes wonderful, sometimes harrowing journey. Surgery is not a guaranteed "cure" for gender dysphoria and indeed many patients well after and recovered from their surgery may see it raise its ugly head from time to time.

It is therefore important for a patient to be kind to themselves and regularly take stock and be proud of all the progress they have made becoming their authentic selves.

About the Authors

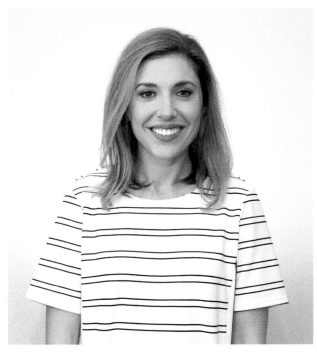

Figure 161 Vanessa de la Llama LMHC

Vanessa de la Llama (she/her) is a Licensed Mental Health Counselor who specializes in working with adolescents and young adults. Vanessa obtained her master's degree in Mental Health Counseling from Nova Southeastern University, and a master's degree in Communications from Florida International University. She completed her clinical internship at Larkin Community Hospital, working with inpatient, Partial Hospitalization Programs (PHP) and Intensive Outpatient Programs (IOP) patients with severe and recurring mental health issues such as depression, anxiety, bipolar, schizophrenia and personality disorders. Vanessa has extensive clinical training and research in child/adolescent psychotherapy, family therapy, and group therapy. Vanessa currently specializes in working with LGBTQ youth, especially Trans. She is currently aligned with WPATH, ACA, and local groups such as Yes! Institute & SunServe. She is fluent in both English and Spanish.

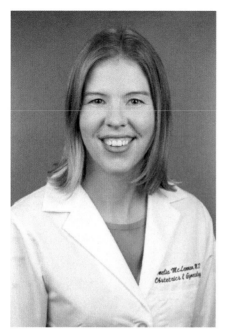

Figure 162 Dr Amy McLennan

Dr. Amy McLennan (she/ her) is a Maternal Fetal Medicine specialist offering care for women with a range of high-risk medical, surgical, and fetal conditions during pregnancy.

She is a co-director of the UC Davis Fetal Care and Treatment Center where she performs in-utero fetal procedures along with a team of specialists including pediatric surgery and cardiology.

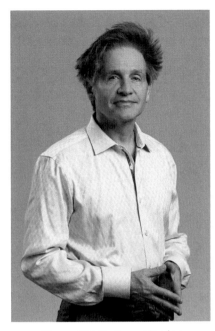

Figure 163 Dr Barry Eppley

Dr. Barry Eppley (he/ his) is one of the United States' most extensively trained and unique plastic surgeons. Dr. Eppley is both a licensed physician and dentist, and is board certified in the specialties of Plastic and Reconstructive Surgery as well as Oral and Maxillofacial Surgery.

He possesses a wealth of international experience in the investigation and development of numerous technologic advances in plastic surgery and has been awarded ten U.S. and international patents on biomedical technologies. His research and clinical efforts have resulted in a large number of contributions to surgical literature with over 250 journal articles and 35 book chapters.

As a plastic surgeon, Dr. Eppley's background and diverse wealth of experience allows him to offer patients an extensive choice of procedures including craniofacial, maxillofacial and all aesthetic facial and body surgeries. As a result of his training background and experience, he is considered the world's foremost authority in the highly technical field of custom facial implants and is responsible for the development of the field of aesthetic skull reshaping.

Dr. Eppley bases his international private plastic surgery practice in the central US in Carmel, Indiana and has developed a uniquely diverse aesthetic practice, with patients traveling to his clinic from all over US, and from 67 other countries as of this writing.

He continues to redefine the field of facial reshaping surgery with the introduction of new facial masculinization and feminization techniques.

For more information please visit:

Eppleyplasticsurgery.com

Eppleycustomfacialimplants.com

Skullreshaping.com

Exploreplasticsurgery.com

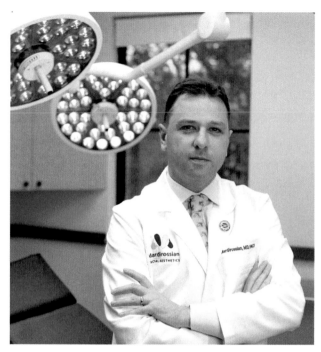

Figure 169 Dr Vartan Mardirossian

Dr. Vartan Mardirossian (he/ his) is double board-certified in both Facial Plastic Surgery and Head and Neck Surgery and has authored many studies on pivotal topics within the realm of Facial Plastic Surgery. He is an Assistant Professor of Facial Plastic and Reconstructive Surgery and Otolaryngology at Florida Atlantic University and a consultant of Facial Plastic and Head and Neck Surgery at Jupiter Medical Center.

He received his undergraduate and medical degrees from the University of Padua in Italy, where he graduated Summa cum Laude in 2000. Dr. Mardirossian completed his Residency in Head and Neck Surgery in Padua, Italy and moved to Boston where he performed research at the Massachusetts Institute of Technology.

Later, he completed an internship in General Surgery, followed by a residency in Otolaryngology – Head and Neck Surgery at Boston University. Further advanced training was obtained with fellowship in Facial Plastic and Reconstructive Surgery through Boston University with world-renowned facial plastic surgeon, Dr. Spiegel.

He currently devotes his practice to facial plastic surgery, facial feminization (FFS) surgery, and vocal feminization surgeries. Vartan Mardirossian MD FACS

Mardirosian Facial Aesthetics

Jupiter, FL

www.palmbeachplastics.com

Genital Gender Affirming Team - OHSU Transgender Health Program

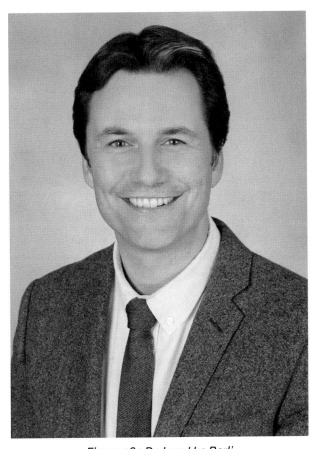

Figure 164 Dr Jens Urs Berli

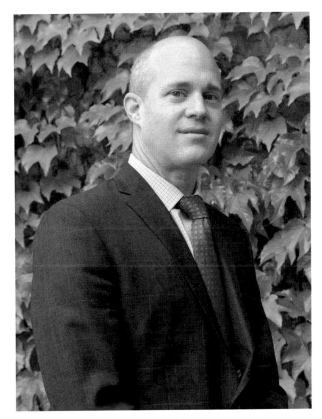

Figure 165 Dr Daniel Dugi

Jens Urs Berli (he/his) is a Swiss/ Danish Associate Professor and Gender Surgeon at Oregon Health & Science University in Portland Oregon. He is particularly passionate about phalloplasty and has lectured and written extensively on the importance for both surgeon and patient to understand all the options that are available for any given individual.

Daniel Dugi (he/his) is a reconstructive urologist and co-founder of Oregon Health & Science University's Transgender Health Program. His practice is dedicated to gender-affirming genital surgery.

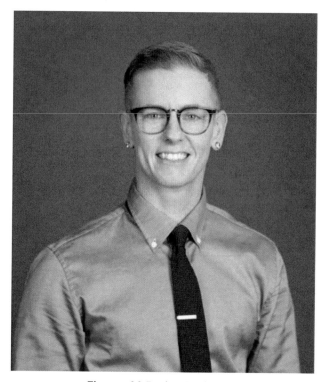

Figure 166 Dorian Scull PA-C

Dorian Scull (he/they) is a physician assistant who works in outpatient gender-affirming surgical urology at OHSU since November 2019. They are passionate about improving the health outcomes of the transgender community through providing competent, gender-affirming, trauma-informed care and training future medical providers to do the same

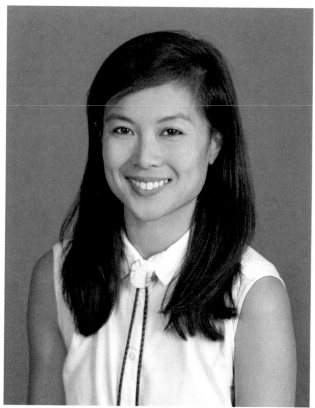

Figure 167 Dr Geolani W. Dy

Geolani W. Dy, MD (she/her) is an Assistant Professor in the Department of Urology and the Transgender Health Program at Oregon Health & Science University. Dr. Dy underwent training in urologic surgery at the University of Washington and completed her fellowship in gender-affirming surgery at New York University. She is passionate about multi-disciplinary collaboration as a pathway for improving trans health outcomes and is devoted to centering patient and community voices in research on gender-affirming surgery.

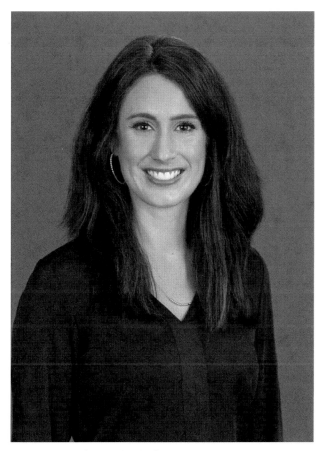

Figure 168 Carley Putnam, PA-C

Carley Putnam (she/her) is a physician assistant who works in gender-affirming plastic surgery at Oregon Health & Science University. She strives to create a comfortable environment for her patients, helping them to plan and prepare for their surgical journey, and ultimately celebrating outcomes all while learning and adapting to the ever-evolving pathway of care for the population which she provides for.

Index

Made in the USA
Las Vegas, NV
10 June 2021